To our friends, family, and colleagues who have patiently endured our lifelong devotion to this medicine.

To our patients, whose trust allows us to do this work.

And to our teachers, and the generations who carried this medicine before them, whose presence endures wherever its principles are brought to life. The credit for the ideas of this book goes to our teachers. Any errors are our own.

A Perspective from Dr. Jordan Barber

One of the central challenges of practicing Chinese medicine today is the contrast between the medicine itself and the pace of modern life. Chinese medicine developed in a world that moved slowly, where observation, reflection, and continuity of care were possible. Modern healthcare, by contrast, often demands speed, efficiency, and brief encounters. This tension shapes both how the medicine is practiced and how it is understood.

When Dr. Peter Caron and I began discussing the possibility of writing a book together, we were trying to address a gap we had both encountered repeatedly. It appeared in two places. The first was in how we explain our work to patients. Much of the reasoning behind what a clinician is doing unfolds over time during treatment, and while pieces of it are shared during visits, there is rarely enough time to explain the underlying logic in a clear and coherent way.

The second place we saw this gap was within acupuncture education itself. Students are exposed to the concepts that form the foundation of clinical reasoning, but they are often encountered in [illegible] ey appear across different courses, different teachers, [illegible] moments in training. Rarely are they presented directly and cohesively as the way one actually learns to think as a clinician within the framework of Chinese medicine.

Our intention in writing this book was simply to make that way of thinking explicit. What we did not expect was that, by the time we finished, the book would feel unusually relevant to the present moment. Medicine is entering a period of rapid technological transformation, particularly with the emergence of artificial intelligence in clinical settings. While tools will continue to evolve, and many aspects of medicine will inevitably change, the core of clinical practice remains something far more difficult to replicate.

Within these pages is an attempt to articulate that core. Techniques, technologies, and systems of documentation will always progress, and they should. Yet the essence of clinical work lies in perception, judgment, and the subtle forms of communication that occur between clinician and patient. These elements cannot be reduced to algorithms.

I am proud of the work that became this book. My hope is that it helps patients better understand the reasoning behind their care, helps students grasp the deeper structure of the medicine they are learning, and reminds practitioners across all fields of medicine that the heart of clinical practice remains profoundly human.

A Perspective from Dr. Peter Caron

I have been practicing Chinese medicine for long enough that certain conversations have become familiar. A patient recovers — sometimes dramatically, sometimes from something that had resisted every prior intervention — and looks at me with a mixture of gratitude and bewilderment. Something magical must have happened. I understand the impulse. When the results outpace the explanation you've been given, when you don't have a rational framework of explanation, what is left except the supernatural?

While understandable, this interpretation is the wrong one, and its prevalence has cost this medicine dearly.

A significant tradition within Chinese medicine has leaned into that mysticism — framing the work in the language of energy, spirit, and cosmic correspondence. The best parts of this reflect genuine philosophical depth, and these ideas can provide surprising results. But much of it has become a barrier: to critical thinking, to clinical rigor, and to the physicians, researchers, and patients who might otherwise take this medicine seriously. When we reach for the ineffable to explain what we do, we trade precision for atmosphere. We make ourselves easy to dismiss.

This book is a direct response to that tradition.

Over the course of more than twenty thousand patient treatments, years of teaching at the graduate level, two years of clinical aid work in rural Guatemala through Global Healthworks Foundation, and building the American Acupuncture Guild as a continuing education platform for practicing clinicians, I have developed a way of explaining this medicine that does not require anyone to suspend their critical faculties. The results I see clinically — and that any well-trained practitioner should be able to reproduce — are not magical. They are the logical output of a coherent clinical framework applied skillfully to a complex system. They have been reproducible and teachable for thousands of years. That continuity is not mysticism. It is the strongest argument for the framework's validity.

The greatest challenge in teaching new acupuncturists is not the volume of material. It is orientation. When confronted with a genuinely different way of thinking, the mind reaches for familiar maps. The discomfort of uncertainty gets traded for the false comfort of analogy. The result is a practitioner who has learned the terminology without acquiring the way of thinking, which is a little like memorizing a city's street names without understanding how to traverse the terrain.

Most of what I teach in the first year is not technique. It is how to think. How to read a body as a system under load rather than a collection of parts with separate complaints. How to find the pattern underneath the symptoms. How to act with precision in the absence of certainty.

That is what this book contains.

My colleague and co-author, Jordan Barber, and I have written it for our patients and medical colleagues who are both bought in and baffled. For empirical reasons, they use and refer to our services, but experience cognitive dissonance about how these empirical results are possible. As you read our text, I hope you see the logical framework we use every day to help people not only recover from disease, but to have better lives.

Everything in here is teachable. None of it requires sleight of hand. And the thinking, once acquired, belongs to anyone willing to learn it.

1

How Chinese Medicine Thinks

People usually come to Chinese medicine the same way they come to any medicine: something isn't working. A symptom won't leave. A diagnosis explains the label but not the lived experience. Tests are "normal," but life isn't. Or the opposite—tests are abnormal, and the treatments are technically correct, yet the body doesn't seem to be getting the message.

By the time most patients—or practitioners—start taking Chinese medicine seriously, they've already learned an uncomfortable truth: the body isn't a machine that breaks in one place and gets fixed in one place. It's closer to a weather system. Patterns form, intensify, shift, and sometimes resolve. A small change can ripple outward. A big intervention can do surprisingly little. And chronic problems have a way of becoming their own ecosystems.

When people think of Chinese Medicine, they think of a set of techniques: needles, herbs, maybe cupping. That's not wrong, but it misses the deeper point. Chinese medicine is a way of thinking clinically. It's a style of reasoning that treats the body as a self-regulating ecosystem—one that can become trapped in loops, pulled off course by stressors, and restored not only by "fighting disease," but by helping the system remember how to adapt again.

If you only take one thing from this chapter, let it be this: Chinese medicine is less interested in what something *is* than in what it is *doing*—and what it is making everything else do in response.

THE BODY AS A SELF-REGULATING ECOSYSTEM

When you walk into a forest, you can't understand what's happening by staring at one leaf. You have to notice relationships: soil, water, sunlight, temperature, microbial life, seasons, and time. A tree isn't just a tree. It's a participant in a dynamic network—responding to, compensating for, and shaping its environment.

Chinese medicine similarly views the human body not as a collection of parts, but as a living ecology of interacting processes: circulation, digestion, sleep, hormonal rhythms, immune surveillance, emotional regulation, thermoregulation, and repair mechanisms. These processes are not separate. They talk to each other constantly.

This communication-based perspective matters because many of the most frustrating health problems are not "broken parts." They're patterns of adaptation that have become expensive.

Take something common: insomnia. The reductionist question is, "What causes insomnia?" and the implied answer is, "One thing, which we should identify and remove." But in real life, insomnia often emerges from a mesh of interacting influences: stress, blood sugar swings, inflammatory load, hormonal transitions, rumination, medication effects, alcohol, post-viral dysregulation, and/or chronic pain. And once insomnia becomes chronic, it starts to change everything else: cortisol rhythm, appetite signaling, mood, immune tone, and pain sensitivity. At that point, it isn't just a symptom. It's a driver.

Chinese medicine asks: *What is the pattern of relationships that produces this?* What are the forces involved, and how is the system trying—and failing—to regulate them?

When we say "ecosystem," we also mean something else: ecosystems self-correct until they can't. They have resilience—then they lose it. They can absorb stress—then they cross a threshold, and suddenly everything looks unstable.

Chinese medicine's perspective emphasizes noticing thresholds and restoring resilience.

THINKING IN SYSTEMS, NOT PARTS

Modern anatomy is miraculous. Surgery saves lives. Imaging can reveal what no hand could palpate. But clinical reasoning can become distorted when our map of the body is mostly structural: organs and tissues as separate objects with distinct specialties.

Chinese medicine uses a different kind of map: functional networks.

In our clinics, you'll hear words like *Liver*, *Spleen*, *Kidney*, *Heart*. To a modern ear, those sound like organs. But in Chinese medicine, these are better understood as *systems of function*—clusters of physiological tasks that tend to rise and fall together.

Thinking in networks can be confusing at first, and it's also where Chinese medicine gains a lot of its power. Because chronic illness often isn't localized. It comes from an issue distributed across these very networks.

A patient might come in with migraines, PMS, reflux, tight shoulders, and a tendency to wake at 3 a.m. A structural lens might scatter this across neurology, gynecology, gastroenterology, orthopedics, and sleep medicine. Each specialty might make a reasonable argument, leaving the patient with a handful of partial explanations.

A systems lens asks: *What single disruption could plausibly generate all of these at once?* Not a single cause in the simplistic sense, but a coherent functional pattern.

In Chinese medicine, these relationships are *patterns*, and when we talk clinically, we discuss treatment strategies for patterns. Pattern recognition isn't mystical. It's a disciplined way of noticing repeated clusters: what tends to co-occur, what triggers what, what relieves what, what follows what.

It's also why two people can have the same diagnosis and receive different treatments in Chinese medicine—because their systems arise from different patterns.

FUNCTION PRECEDES STRUCTURE

One of the most clinically useful assumptions in Chinese medicine is that function tends to shift before structure does.

In plain language, the body starts behaving differently before it starts looking different on a scan.

Sometimes, structure clearly comes first—acute trauma, a fracture, an infection that destroys tissue. But in many chronic conditions, especially those driven by stress physiology, inflammation, metabolic drift, or post-viral dysregulation, the earliest changes are functional: sleep becomes lighter, digestion becomes less tolerant, temperature regulation becomes erratic, mood becomes more reactive, cycles shift, and recovery slows down.

If you wait until the structure changes enough to be obvious—until labs flag, imaging shows degeneration, or pathology declares itself—you've often missed years of early leverage.

Chinese medicine is comfortable working in that earlier territory, where the signs are subtle, and the system is compensating. That's not because it rejects modern testing; it's because it takes the patient's lived pattern seriously even when the tests are "fine." This approach is often called preventative medicine, but it's really early detection.

Clinically, this is one of the most relieving moments for patients: when someone treats their experience as real data rather than something fuzzy and subjective without value.

QI: ORGANIZED ACTIVITY, NOT A SUBSTANCE

If there's one word that attracts misunderstanding, it's *Qi*.

People tend to imagine Qi as a mystical vapor, a magical energy that you either "have" or you don't. Others dismiss it as pre-scientific nonsense. Both reactions miss what the term is doing.

In Chinese medicine, Qi is *organized activity*—the capacity of the body to coordinate function coherently.

That includes things we can measure (metabolic activity, neural signaling, circulation, motility, immune response) and things we experience (alertness, stamina, warmth, appetite, the ability to initiate action and complete it). Qi is not a single thing. It's a category word for a *function that is alive, directed, and coherent.*

When Qi is sufficient and well-regulated, systems communicate. Digestion transforms food into usable fuel. Blood circulates to the periphery. Sleep comes when it's time to sleep. Stress responses turn on when needed, then turn off. The body doesn't just react—it adjusts.

When Qi is disordered, it tends to show up as either:

- **Not enough coordinated activity** (fatigue, weakness, poor recovery, spontaneous sweating, shortness of breath, low appetite, brain fog), or

- **Poorly regulated activity** (tension, spasms, reflux, irritability, palpitations, insomnia, headaches), or

- **Misplaced activity** (things moving the wrong way: nausea, hiccups, coughing, flushing, anxiety surges), or

- **Stuck activity** (pain, distension, mood constraint, irregular cycles).

Notice that none of these require believing in a mysterious substance, but rather noticing patterns of function.

Qi is a heuristic model, a practical clinical idea: it gives you language for *how the body is behaving as a coordinated whole*, not just what part hurts.

YIN AND YANG: RELATIONAL PROCESSES, NOT OPPOSING FORCES

At first, Yin and Yang are like a cartoon: dark/light, cold/hot, feminine/masculine, two opposing forces locked in eternal combat.

That version is memorable. It's also clinically shallow.

In the clinic, Yin and Yang are *relational processes*—the way the body organizes opposites that depend on each other.

A simple example: activity and rest. If you push activity without rest, the system overheats, frays, and becomes reactive. If you rest without meaningful activity, the system stagnates, becomes dull, and loses tone. Health isn't choosing one side. It's maintaining a dynamic relationship between them.

Yin tends to describe substance, cooling, moistening, anchoring, storing, settling, and restoring. Yang tends to describe movement, warming, mobilization, transformation, defense, and activation.

But the key is their relationship:

- Yin without Yang becomes inert.
- Yang without Yin becomes uncontained.
- Yin and Yang aren't enemies; they're mutual requirements.

Clinically, this matters because many chronic conditions are not "too much" or "too little" in a simple way. They're *imbalanced relationships*.

A person can be exhausted (low functional reserve) and simultaneously wired (excess sympathetic activation). They can have cold hands and feet, but feel heat in their face at night. They can be depressed and anxious. They can have low appetite but intense cravings. The body can be conserving in one area and overreacting in another.

Yin–Yang thinking is not about forcing a label. It's about

tracking *where regulation has become skewed* and what the system is doing to compensate for it.

HEALTH AS ADAPTABILITY, NOT THE ABSENCE OF DISEASE

Most people define health as "nothing wrong." No symptoms, no diagnosis, normal labs.

But the lived reality is more subtle. Plenty of people have "normal" labs while feeling brittle—one bad night of sleep and everything collapses. Others have a diagnosis yet live with stability, energy, and resilience.

Chinese medicine quietly uses a different definition: health is *adaptability*.

Adaptability means:

- You can handle stress and recover.
- You can travel, eat differently, miss a night of sleep, catch a mild cold, and bounce back.
- You can feel emotions without being hijacked by them.
- Your cycles—sleep, digestion, mood, temperature—have rhythm and flexibility.

From this perspective, chronic illness often looks like a loss of options. The system narrows. It becomes reactive. It stops adapting and starts bracing.

A useful clinical question becomes: *Where is the body rigid?* Where has it lost flexibility? That rigidity might show up as muscle tension, yes—but also as rigid sleep timing, rigid dietary requirements, rigid mood loops, rigid inflammatory reactions, rigid hormone patterns.

Treatment then aims not only to reduce symptoms, but to restore the system's ability to change state without crashing.

THE RESPONSE MATTERS AS MUCH AS THE DISEASE

One of the most important shifts Chinese medicine offers is this: the body's response can be as clinically significant as the trigger.

Two people catch the same virus. One has a mild fever for a day and moves on. The other develops a lingering cough, fatigue, palpitations, brain fog, and months of dysregulation. Two people experience the same stressor. One becomes focused and productive; the other spirals into insomnia and digestive upset.

The difference is not moral. It's regulatory capacity.

Modern medicine is very good at identifying external threats: pathogens, allergens, tumors, toxins. Chinese medicine focuses on the internal terrain: *How is the system responding? What kind of response is this body inclined to produce?*

The response is not an either/or question. It's both. You need to know what you're dealing with—and you need to understand why this body is having *this* reaction.

In practice, this is why Chinese medicine can be useful even when the biomedical diagnosis is clear. The diagnosis names the category; the pattern describes the lived physiology.

WHY CHINESE MEDICINE AVOIDS SINGLE-CAUSE EXPLANATIONS

Patients often want a clean answer: "What caused this?" Practitioners want it too, even if we pretend otherwise. This desire is natural. A single cause feels solvable. It promises control.

But in complex biology, single-cause stories are often fictions we tell to make uncertainty tolerable.

Chinese medicine doesn't avoid causality—it avoids simplistic causality. It assumes that most chronic conditions arise from *multiple interacting influences* over time, shaped by constitution, environment, habits, emotional load, infections, injuries, reproductive history, and the accumulation of small imbalances.

A single-cause explanation might be true in acute situations: food poisoning from a specific meal, an asthma attack triggered by a cat, a fracture from a fall. But chronic problems are rarely that clean.

And here's the part that matters clinically: even if you find the original trigger, the body may no longer be responding to the trigger. It may be responding to the *new pattern* that formed afterward.

Think of a microphone that squeals with feedback. The original sound could have been a whisper, a cough, a single note. But once the loop is established, the loop becomes the problem. You don't fix it by blaming the whisper. You fix it by changing the system conditions that allow the loop to self-amplify.

Chinese medicine is a feedback-oriented medicine.

FEEDBACK LOOPS, AND THE SECOND- AND THIRD-ORDER EFFECTS

Reductionist thinking tends to focus on first-order effects: A causes B. Treat A, and B improves.

Systems thinking asks: What does B do next? What does the treatment do next? What does the compensation do next?

Second- and third-order effects are where chronic illness often lives.

Example 1: Stress → Digestion → Sleep → Stress (Loop)

- Stress increases sympathetic tone.
- Sympathetic tone reduces digestive motility and secretion.
- Digestion becomes sluggish or reactive; blood sugar becomes less stable.
- Sleep becomes lighter or broken.

- Poor sleep increases cortisol dysregulation and emotional reactivity.
- Stress becomes easier to trigger and harder to discharge.

Now the symptom list can look unrelated—bloating, reflux, insomnia, anxiety, fatigue—but the system is stuck in a loop. Treating only the reflux may help temporarily, but the loop keeps generating reflux.

Chinese medicine would ask: Where can we interrupt the loop? Sometimes the best entry point is to calm the nervous system and anchor sleep. Sometimes it's about supporting digestive function so the body doesn't get pushed into a stress response by its own instability.

Example 2: Pain → Guarding → Stagnation → More Pain (Loop)

- An injury or inflammation produces pain.
- The bodyguards: muscles tighten, movement becomes restricted.
- Circulation decreases; local tissues become more ischemic and sensitized.
- The nervous system becomes more vigilant.
- Pain increases, and the guarding intensifies.

In Chinese medicine language, you might hear terms like "stagnation" or "constraint." These aren't metaphors. They are functional descriptions of reduced movement and impaired regulation—often very literal in the tissues and the nervous system.

Example 3: "Cold" Patterns and Compensatory Heat (Second-Order)

Some patients present with an interesting mix: cold limbs, low appetite, fatigue, frequent urination—yet also flushing, hot sensations at night, or anxiety spikes. A simplistic view might argue, "Are they cold or hot? Pick one."

But clinically, this can reflect a system with low foundational warmth and circulation (a Yang insufficiency, in Chinese terms) that produces *secondary heat* because regulation is unstable: the body can't distribute warmth smoothly, so it surges upward or appears as false heat when the system pushes past its resiliency.

If you only "clear heat," you can worsen the underlying weakness. If you only "warm," you can aggravate the flares. The art is understanding the *relationship* and choosing interventions that restore regulation rather than chasing the loudest symptom.

Example 4: Over-suppression as a Third-Order Problem

This one is uncomfortable, but important. Sometimes a symptom is not the disease—it's the body's attempt to solve a problem.

Diarrhea can be the body's way of evacuating irritation. A fever can be a coordinated immune strategy. Inflammation can be protective, at least initially.

If you suppress the response without understanding why it's happening, you might get a short-term win and a long-term complication: the symptom changes form, goes deeper, becomes chronic, or rebounds stronger. Third-order thinking isn't an argument against symptom relief. It's an argument for respecting the logic of the response.

Chinese medicine trains you to ask: *What is this symptom trying to accomplish?* Even when it's maladaptive, it usually began as an intelligent attempt.

WHY REDUCTIONISM STRUGGLES IN CHRONIC AND COMPLEX CONDITIONS

Reductionism is not stupid. It's powerful. It's how we learned what insulin does, how bacteria cause pneumonia, and how anticoagulants prevent stroke.

But reductionism struggles when:

1. **There are multiple interacting variables**, none of which is sufficient on its own.

2. **The system adapts to the intervention**, creating new dynamics.

3. **The problem is distributed**, not localized.

4. **The timeline is long**, with phases that change over years.

5. **The outcome depends on context**, like sleep, relationships, and stress load—factors that are real physiology but hard to isolate.

Chronic illness often involves all five.

A patient with IBS, migraines, anxiety, and eczema is not a puzzle that yields to one missing piece. You can find food sensitivities, inflammatory markers, microbiome changes, stressors, trauma history, hormonal shifts—and still not have the satisfying "root cause" moment.

Chinese medicine's advantage is not that it knows the magical root. It's that it doesn't require one. It can still act clinically by working with patterns of regulation: supporting what's weak, venting what's stuck, cooling what's inflamed, warming what's underactive, harmonizing what's discordant.

It's a different kind of precision—less about a single target and more about shifting the behavior of the whole system.

THE CHALLENGE OF MULTI-FACTOR CAUSAL MAPS

Of course, systems thinking has its own problem: it can become vague. If everything affects everything, how do you decide what to do Monday at 10 a.m. when a real person is sitting in front of you?

This is where Chinese medicine earns its keep—not in theory, but in method.

A skilled clinician builds a causal map without pretending it's complete. You listen for key nodes—places where many lines converge. You look for "driver" patterns rather than "passenger" symptoms. You test hypotheses through treatment: if I move this lever, does the whole system shift?

It's not guesswork, but it is probabilistic. It's closer to navigation than to geometry.

You might suspect, for example, that a patient's chronic headaches are driven less by the head and more by:

- sleep rhythm instability,
- neck and rib cage restriction affecting breathing mechanics,
- digestive stagnation generating upward pressure,
- long-term jaw clenching from sympathetic dominance,
- or menstrual cycle dynamics.

All of those could be true. The clinical art is choosing an entry point that is safe, effective, and responsive—and then watching what changes.

In other words, Chinese medicine is not anti-causal. It is *multi-causal with prioritization.*

SCIENCE AND MODERN RESEARCH: ONE TOOL AMONG MANY

There's a stereotype that Chinese medicine is "ancient wisdom" floating above evidence, and another stereotype that it's "unscientific," unless it translates into biomedical terms.

Both stereotypes flatten reality.

In practice, modern research is one tool among many that clinicians use to make decisions. It can inform safety, dosing, mechanism hypotheses, and probability. It can help us avoid errors and update older assumptions. It can point to promising interventions and warn us away from harmful ones.

But science, as usually practiced, also has limits:

- Research often isolates variables that are inseparable in real life.
- Many studies are short-term, while chronic illness is long-term.
- Outcomes measured in trials may not align with what matters to patients (resilience, sleep quality, digestive tolerance, relapse frequency).
- Individual variability gets averaged out, even when it's the point.

Chinese medicine, done well, is not in competition with science. It simply refuses to pretend that science is the only way to know what is happening in a complex individual system.

The clinic is also a kind of laboratory—messy, uncontrolled, ethically constrained, but rich in pattern information. You treat, you observe, you adjust. You learn what tends to follow what.

A mature approach holds both respect for research and respect for lived physiology.

CHINESE MEDICINE AS MACRO-LEVEL POETRY—OFTEN CONFIRMED BY MICRO-LEVEL SCIENCE

Chinese medicine uses language that can sound poetic: wind, dampness, heat, cold, dryness, and fire. At first glance, this appears to be a metaphor. Sometimes it is a metaphor. But often it's closer to a macro-level functional description—an attempt to name patterns that are real but not easily captured by a single biomarker.

For example:

- **"Dampness"** often corresponds to a cluster of signs: heaviness, swelling, sluggish digestion, sticky stools, foggy thinking, and a greasy tongue coat. Micro-level correlates might include inflammatory cytokines, altered microbiota, impaired lymphatic flow, insulin resistance, or edema mechanisms—depending on the person. The Chinese term doesn't replace these. It groups the *felt and observed patterns* in a way that guides treatment.
- **"Heat"** describes patterns like inflammation, redness, irritability, thirst, burning sensations, rapid pulse, and restless sleep. Micro-level correlates might include increased sympathetic tone, inflammatory signaling, histamine activity, hormonal shifts, or infection-driven immune activation.
- **"Wind"** is used for movement and changeability: tremors, spasms, dizziness, sudden itching, symptoms that shift quickly. A modern lens might look at neurological excitability, vestibular dysfunction, mast cell activation, or dysautonomia.

The point is not to force equivalence. The point is that the macro-level pattern is clinically actionable.

This is why Chinese medicine can feel strange and yet strangely accurate. It's describing the body at the level where patterns are experienced and treated, not at the level of isolated mechanisms.

When micro-level science validates these patterns, it's satisfying—but it isn't required for the pattern to be clinically useful. And when micro-level science *contradicts* a traditional assumption, a good clinician updates rather than clings.

Chinese medicine at its best is not nostalgia. It's a disciplined language for complexity.

A DIFFERENT KIND OF CLINICAL PRECISION

So what does it mean, practically, to "think like Chinese medicine"?

It means you're always asking questions that point toward regulation:

- What is the body trying to do?
- What is it failing to do?
- What is it doing too much of, too often, or in the wrong place?
- What compensations are currently keeping the person functional—and what are those compensations costing?
- What patterns repeat across different systems?
- What happens when we nudge the system—does it soften, stabilize, or resist?

It also means you stop treating symptoms as isolated events and start treating them as messages from a network.

That shift can feel unsettling, because it removes the false comfort of simple causes. But it also opens something more useful: a path forward even when the case is complex.

If the body is a self-regulating ecosystem, then healing isn't always about force. Often it's about restoring conditions under which regulation becomes possible again: better circulation, better sleep rhythm, better digestion, steadier emotional processing, and less internal friction. Not perfection—adaptability.

This is the groundwork for everything that follows in this book. We'll talk about the tools—acupuncture, herbs, manual techniques, lifestyle strategies—but the tools only make sense inside the thinking. The medicine isn't the needle. The medicine is the clinical reasoning that tells you where to place it, when to use it, and what kind of change you're actually trying to produce.

In the next chapter, we'll start building the map Chinese medicine uses to track these patterns—how it gathers data from the body, and how that data becomes a treatment strategy rather than a list of disconnected complaints.

2

Where This Medicine Comes From

People often imagine Chinese medicine as something that *descended* —a finished philosophy handed down from antiquity, polished by sages, preserved in amber. That story is tidy. It's also not how medicine is born.

Medicine—any medicine—emerges from three stubborn realities:

1. Bodies get sick in patterns.
2. Someone has to take care of the sick.
3. Communities can't function if too many people are unwell.

Chinese medicine grew inside those realities. It didn't start as "Eastern philosophy." It started as observation: of weather, crops, work, hunger, stress, war, childbirth, aging, and the way certain interventions reliably shifted the course of illness. Over time, those observations hardened into methods—some brilliant, some wrong, many incomplete, all shaped by the constraints of their era.

If you want to understand classical Chinese medicine, it helps to stop asking, "What did the ancients *believe*?" and start asking, "What did they have to *manage*?"

This chapter is about that management: nature, agriculture, governance, and the kind of physician that early China produced. It's also about why the classical texts read the way they do—why they can feel alien if you approach them as philosophy, and why they become startlingly practical when you approach them as clinical records. And finally, it's about how modern standardized TCM was created, what it preserved, what it flattened, and why disagreement among physicians is not an embarrassing flaw in the tradition but one of its core safety features.

NATURE IS THE FIRST TEACHER, BUT NOT IN THE SENTIMENTAL WAY

When modern people hear "observation of nature," they often picture sages watching clouds and writing metaphors about mist becoming dew. That image isn't entirely wrong—it's just incomplete. The most important "nature" in early medicine wasn't a poetic landscape. It was the blunt, repetitive nature of seasons and survival.

If you farm, you learn quickly that the same inputs do not produce the same outputs year-round. You learn that timing matters as much as substance. You learn that damp weather rots grain, that wind dries soil, that early frost changes everything. You learn to read small signs—leaf curl, soil smell, insect behavior—because waiting for certainty is how you lose a harvest.

Now translate that into bodies.

When I sit with a patient, and we're trying to understand why their digestion collapses every spring, or why their insomnia peaks in late summer, or why a skin condition flares with humidity, the logic we're using is not mystical. It's agricultural logic applied to physiology: systems responding to environment, timing, and stress load.

Early Chinese medicine was built in a world where people tracked:

- seasonal changes with obsessive seriousness,
- labor patterns (planting, harvesting, winter storage),
- food availability and food spoilage,
- water quality,
- epidemic waves that followed travel routes and military campaigns.

That's why "wind," "cold," "damp," and "heat" became core medical language. Not because ancient people lacked microscopes, but because they were describing *how illness behaves* in relation to climate and exposure.

"Wind" isn't a poetic word in the clinic. It's a way of naming rapid onset, movement, changeability—symptoms that migrate, tremors that shift, rashes that appear and disappear, pain that moves. "Damp" isn't a vibe; it's a cluster: heaviness, swelling, turbidity, sluggish transformation, sticky stools, weeping skin lesions, recurrent yeast-like patterns, foggy thinking with fatigue. "Cold" and "heat" aren't moral categories; they're functional descriptions of speed, constriction, inflammation, appetite, thirst, restlessness, color, and response to warmth or coolness.

This is the first crucial point: Chinese medical language is not primarily a theory about the universe. It's a shorthand for pattern recognition under real-world constraints.

And those constraints mattered. If you live in a place where winter kills, where famine is a recurring threat, where clean water isn't guaranteed, you get very good at noticing what happens *before* catastrophe. Chinese medicine is full of that kind of noticing.

AGRICULTURE: THE HIDDEN BACKBONE OF CLINICAL THINKING

Agriculture shaped Chinese medicine in ways that are easy to miss if you've only encountered it through modern acupuncture brochures.

1) Food is medicine because food was the baseline intervention

In early societies, the boundary between "food therapy" and "herbal therapy" wasn't clear. Many medicinal substances were also foods, and many foods were evaluated for their physiological effects. When you don't have pharmaceuticals, and when supply chains are unreliable, you treat with what is available and repeatable.

Even now, in our clinics, some of the most meaningful shifts happen when a patient stops unknowingly undermining their treatment every day. Not because I'm moralizing diet, but because physiology is honest: if digestion is weak, if fluids aren't transforming well, if inflammation is constantly fed, no herb formula can fully compensate. Classical medicine never forgot that because it grew inside a food economy.

2) Timing is part of the medicine

Farmers don't ask only *what* to do. They ask *when*. Classical medicine shares that mindset. The seasonal emphasis in the classics isn't decorative. It's an attempt to encode timing into clinical decisions: when sweating is safe, when it's dangerous; when nourishing is appropriate, when it traps pathogens; when "draining" helps, when it weakens.

A simple clinical example: two people can present with the same headache. One needs the surface released—light sweating, gentle movement of constrained circulation. The other needs nourishment and anchoring because the headache is a rebound effect of deficiency and instability. Treat them the same, and you'll help one and harm the other. The classics are obsessed with this difference, and that obsession comes from a world where mistakes cost lives.

3) Storage and spoilage taught clinicians to think about "pathogens" and "accumulation."

Before germ theory, people still knew that rot spreads, that stagnant water breeds trouble, and that certain conditions generate toxicity. Those observations fed into medical concepts of accumulation, turbidity, phlegm, and "heat toxins." Again: not mystical, not modern microbiology either—just careful attention to what tends to happen when things don't move and transform cleanly.

When a patient describes that their body feels "stuck"—swollen, heavy, foggy, chronically congested, always producing mucus, always inflamed after meals—I'm not thinking about a philosophical concept. I'm thinking about transformation and transportation failing, and I'm thinking about how to restore function without collapsing their vitality.

That's agricultural medicine: protect the system that processes inputs and manages waste.

GOVERNANCE: WHY STATES CARE ABOUT MEDICINE

The second overlooked origin point is governance.

A state cares about medicine for the same reason it cares about roads and grain stores: labor and stability. Epidemics disrupt tax revenue, military readiness, and social order. Childbirth outcomes shape the population. Famine and disease travel together. In that context, medicine isn't just personal—it's infrastructure.

This is why, across Chinese history, you see recurring attempts to:

- collect and standardize medical knowledge,
- train court physicians,
- compile formularies,
- respond to epidemics with organized measures,
- regulate dangerous substances.

These weren't always successful, and they weren't purely benevolent. But they shaped what survived.

One consequence is that Chinese medicine developed an unusual relationship with writing. In many cultures, medical knowledge stayed largely oral for long periods. In China, literacy and bureaucracy created a setting where medicine could be debated, compiled, edited, and transmitted through texts—especially among physician-scholars.

That brings us to a crucial figure in the history of Chinese medicine: the physician-scholar.

THE PHYSICIAN-SCHOLAR MODEL: MEDICINE AS AN EXTENSION OF STUDY

When people say "Chinese medicine is scholarly," they sometimes mean "it's theoretical." That's not quite right. The deeper truth is that, in many periods of Chinese history, the people who had the time and training to write were the same people who were steeped in classical learning, ethics, and governance. Some of them became physicians, especially when political careers were blocked or when family circumstances demanded practical skill.

So you get a particular type: a clinician who reads widely, writes case records, debates other doctors through essays, and treats medicine as a craft worthy of serious study.

This matters because it shaped *how* medical knowledge was recorded.

A physician-scholar doesn't just list recipes. They argue. They annotate. They compare interpretations. They write about mistakes. They preserve dissent. They show their reasoning.

In the clinic, this is one of the things I love most about classical medicine: it assumes the clinician is thinking. It doesn't reduce medicine to a checklist. It expects you to develop judgment.

That's also why classical training can feel uncomfortable to modern students. Modern education often rewards correct answers. Classical medicine rewards correct *decisions* in messy conditions—

decisions that require you to tolerate ambiguity and still act responsibly.

WHY THE CLASSICAL TEXTS ARE CLINICAL RECORDS, NOT PHILOSOPHY BOOKS

Many people first encounter Chinese medicine through words like *yin-yang* and *five phases* and assume the classics are metaphysical treatises. Those frameworks are in there, yes. But if you read the major clinical classics closely, the heartbeat of the text is not metaphysics. It's **problem-solving**.

The *Shang Han Lun* (Treatise on Cold Damage, 200AD), for example, is often presented as an "ancient theory" of external infection. But what it really reads like—when you stop trying to turn it into a modern pathology textbook—is a set of tightly organized clinical scenarios:

- Here is what you see.
- Here is what tends to happen next if you do nothing.
- Here is what happens if you treat incorrectly.
- Here is what happens when you treat correctly.
- Here is the formula that matches that pattern.
- Here are the modifications when certain details change.

That is not philosophy. That is a Physician's Desk Reference.

Even the *Huangdi Neijing* (Yellow Emperor's Inner Classic), which contains more cosmological language, is saturated with clinical concerns: how to examine, how to time interventions, how to avoid harming the patient, how emotions and lifestyle disrupt physiology, and what constitutes real skill versus performance.

If you approach these texts as if they are trying to explain the universe, you'll either dismiss them or mythologize them. If you approach them as clinical archives—compressed, sometimes cryptic, occasionally contradictory—you start to see something else: a long conversation among practitioners trying to encode what they learned the hard way.

Why are they so hard to read, then?

Partly because they're written in a different medical culture. But partly because they're written like notes intended for insiders. Classical texts often assume you already have a living teacher and a clinic to test ideas in. They don't hold your hand. They don't always define terms. They rely on shared context.

In other words, they were not written to be "accessible." They were written to be *useful to the initiated.*

And that leads to the next issue: how this medicine is actually transmitted.

LINEAGE TRANSMISSION VS STANDARDIZED EDUCATION

There are two very different ways to transmit a medical system:

1. **Lineage transmission**: apprenticeship, mentorship, direct correction, embodied skills, case-by-case learning.
2. **Standardized education**: curricula, textbooks, exams, uniform terminology, reproducible training pathways.

Most modern people assume standardized education is automatically superior. It isn't. It's superior at certain goals—scale, consistency, baseline safety. But it cannot transmit everything that matters clinically.

What lineage does well

Lineage training—at its best—is not secretive mysticism. It's a close-range clinical formation.

A good mentor doesn't just tell you which points to needle or which formula to give. They train your attention.

They correct the way you take a pulse. They show you what you missed in the patient's voice. They teach you which details are "noise" and which details change the entire direction of treatment.

They transmit timing, dosage sense, and the art of not over-treating.

Most importantly, they teach you how to change your mind when the body responds in an unexpected way.

This is one reason classical case records (*yi'an*) are so valuable. They preserve not only outcomes but also the thought process: why the physician chose one approach, how they adjusted and what they learned.

What standardized education does well

Standardized education creates a floor. It helps prevent dangerous improvisation. It makes sure practitioners share a common vocabulary. It allows medicine to be taught at scale. It supports research and regulation. It creates access.

If you've ever met a brilliant lineage doctor who is also inconsistent, opaque, or cavalier about safety, you understand why societies push toward standardization.

The problem is not that standardization exists. The problem is when standardization is mistaken for the medicine itself.

Because when you flatten a living clinical tradition into a curriculum, you inevitably privilege what is easiest to test and easiest to agree on. You tend to lose:

- the edge cases,
- the dissenting interpretations,
- the high-level pulse and diagnostic nuance,
- the dosage sophistication,
- the "this works but only if you understand when not to use it" kind of knowledge.

You get something teachable. You don't always get something deep. You're not optimizing for physician-scholars, you're optimizing for basic competency and consistency.

This tension between lineage and standardization is not unique to Chinese medicine. But in China, it became historically acute—and it set the stage for the creation of what we now call TCM.

THE HISTORICAL REASONS TCM WAS CREATED (AND THE PROBLEM IT WAS SOLVING)

"TCM" (Traditional Chinese Medicine) sounds like an ancient category. It isn't. It's a modern construction—primarily a mid-20th-century project of consolidation, standardization, and institutional survival.

To understand why it happened, you have to look at the pressures China faced:

- Political upheaval and war,
- The rise of biomedicine and its institutions,
- The need for public health on a massive scale,
- The practical shortage of biomedical doctors,
- The desire to preserve a cultural asset while also modernizing the nation.

Classical medicine existed in many forms—regional schools, family lineages, individual masters, textual traditions, and folk practices. It was powerful, but it wasn't unified. It also wasn't always regulated in a way that a modern state could rely on.

So the state did what states do: it organized.

TCM was built to be teachable in universities, deployable in hospitals, legible to policy, and compatible—at least administratively—with biomedical systems. That meant:

- standard terminology,
- standard pattern categories,
- standardized point prescriptions,
- standardized herb functions and indications,
- standardized textbooks,
- standardized licensing.

This brought real benefits. It protected Chinese medicine from being erased. It created pathways for education and employment. It allowed Chinese medicine to participate in national healthcare. It made research and regulation possible.

But it also created a shadow: the idea that the standardized version is the "real" version, and everything else is either backward, secretive, or irrelevant.

That's where many modern misunderstandings come from. People argue about whether Chinese medicine is "scientific" or "superstitious" without realizing they're often arguing about an educational product—TCM—rather than the broader classical clinical tradition that TCM drew from.

In practice, many excellent clinicians are TCM-trained and also deeply classical in their thinking. And many classical practitioners use standardized tools when appropriate. This isn't a purity contest. It's about recognizing what each system can and cannot carry.

Which raises the question: what is preserved in classical medicine that standardization cannot retain?

WHAT CLASSICAL MEDICINE PRESERVES THAT STANDARDIZATION CAN'T HOLD

Standardization is good at preserving *content*. It is not as good at preserving *judgment*.

Classical medicine preserves certain kinds of clinical intelligence that are difficult to turn into curricula.

1) The primacy of pattern over diagnosis labels

Modern standardized systems tend to reify categories. You learn "Liver qi stagnation" as if it's a stable entity. In real classical practice, patterns are provisional. They are descriptions of a moving target.

Two patients can share a Western diagnosis and require completely different approaches. Two patients can share a TCM pattern label and still require different formulas, timing, and priorities because the label is only a rough map.

Classical medicine holds tightly to this: treat what is happening, not what it is called.

2) Formula thinking as a living language

In many standardized programs, formulas become "for" things. This formula is for headaches; that one is for insomnia. That's a teaching shortcut. It's also a clinical trap.

In classical practice, formulas are more like sentences than pills. Their structure matters. Their internal logic matters. You learn what each herb is doing in *that particular combination* and how the formula behaves when you adjust it.

This is why two practitioners can treat the same patient with different formulas and both be right—if their reasoning is sound and their follow-up is sharp. It's also why copying a formula without understanding can fail dramatically.

3) The art of dosage and the ethics of force

Standardization tends to default to moderate, safe dosing ranges and conservative approaches—again, for good reasons. But classical medicine includes a wide range of forces: gentle nudges, strong pivots, rescue interventions, and slow rebuilding.

In the classics, you see repeated warnings about over-treating—about sweating too much, purging too much, warming too much, tonifying too early, dispersing when the system is already collapsed.

This is not theoretical. It's the ethical core of medicine: **don't show off; don't force the body; don't mistake intensity for effectiveness.**

You can't fully standardize that. You have to develop it by watching bodies respond.

4) Diagnostic skill as an embodied craft

Pulse diagnosis, tongue observation, listening, smelling, palpation, the ability to detect subtle shifts over time—these are not fully transmissible through textbooks. They require correction by a skilled eye and hand.

A modern program can teach the basics. But the high-level skill—the kind that changes outcomes in complex chronic illness—usually comes from prolonged mentorship and extensive clinical feedback.

5) Permission to revise the model when the patient doesn't match it

This one is easy to overlook: classical medicine is comfortable with being incomplete.

The classics preserve arguments, alternatives, and exceptions. Standardization tends to smooth those out. It says, "Here are the categories." Classical medicine says, "Here is what often works—until it doesn't. Then pay attention."

That is not a flaw. That is an adaptive trait that acknowledges complexity and nuance.

Which brings us to something that confuses modern readers: the tradition contains disagreement—sometimes sharp disagreement. And that disagreement is not a failure of coherence. It's part of how the medicine stays alive.

WHY DISAGREEMENT AMONG PHYSICIANS IS A FEATURE, NOT A FLAW

A common critique goes like this: "If Chinese medicine were real, practitioners would agree. But one doctor says my condition is damp-heat, another says it's yin deficiency. So it must be subjective."

The critique feels reasonable—until you remember that disagreement exists in every living medical system. Ask three orthopedic surgeons about a borderline back surgery case. Ask two psychiatrists about a complex medication plan. Ask five internists about the best first-line approach for mild hypertension in a particular patient with unusual constraints. You'll get variance.

The question isn't whether disagreement exists. The question is: **what kind of disagreement is it, and what contains it?**

In good Chinese medicine, disagreement is often one of three things:

1) Different prioritizations of the same complex reality

Complex cases are layered. A patient can have a genuine deficiency and a genuine excess at the same time. They can have constraints in one system and collapse in another. They can have heat above and cold below. They can have inflammation from stagnation and fatigue from depletion.

One practitioner might prioritize clearing what is stuck because it is the most immediate driver of symptoms. Another might prioritize stabilizing the foundation because the patient cannot tolerate clearing. If both are attentive and follow the response, both approaches can be legitimate.

This is not relativism. It's triage.

2) Different lineages emphasize different diagnostic anchors

Some lineages lean heavily on pulse. Some on abdominal diagnosis. Some on formula families from specific texts. Some on five-phase constitutional thinking. These anchors shape how a practitioner organizes the data.

If the practitioner is well-trained, their anchor doesn't blind them—it disciplines them. But it can lead to different languages and different starting points.

What matters is not whether everyone uses the same words. What matters is whether the intervention helps, whether it is adjusted intelligently, and whether it avoids predictable harm.

3) Disagreement functions as a check against dogma

The tradition's internal pluralism prevents it from being fully captured by a single ideology. If one school becomes too rigid, another school points out what it's missing. If one approach becomes fashionable, another reminds us of the edge cases where it fails.

In that sense, disagreement is part of the quality-control system.

I've had patients come in after being told, with absolute certainty, that they must avoid all warming herbs forever because they are "already hot." Then I examine them: cold limbs, weak digestion, fatigue that improves with warmth, a tongue that shows pale swelling, a pulse that lacks strength. The "heat" is real—but it may be a false heat floating above a cold foundation, or a constrained heat from stagnation rather than robust excess.

If the practitioner cannot imagine that possibility, the patient gets trapped in a treatment that fits a label rather than a body.

Disagreement, when grounded in skill, is one way the medicine protects itself from that trap.

THE QUIET THREAD RUNNING THROUGH ALL OF THIS: CLINICAL REALITY

If you step back, a consistent thread appears.

Chinese medicine did not originate as an abstract worldview. It emerged from:

- people watching how bodies respond to seasons, food, labor, and stress,
- physicians recording what worked and what backfired,
- scholar-clinicians debating methods through texts and case records,
- governments attempting to preserve and deploy medical capacity at scale.

That history created two parallel inheritances:

1. a **classical** inheritance: textured, argumentative, hard to standardize, rich in clinical subtlety;
2. a **modern standardized** inheritance (TCM): teachable, scalable, researchable, regulated, often simplified.

Both are real—both matter. The trouble comes when we confuse one for the other, or when we demand that a living clinical art behave like a single-author manual.

The patient in front of you is not a standardized object. They are a moving ecosystem—one that responds, adapts, resists, surprises you, and sometimes teaches you something you didn't know you needed to learn. As I mentioned earlier in this book, the clinic is its own kind of laboratory—messy, ethically constrained, but filled with pattern information. Classical medicine grew up inside that kind of lab for centuries.

So if the tradition feels less like a cathedral of fixed doctrine and more like a crowded marketplace of experienced voices—that's because it is.

And that's not a reason to distrust it.

It's a reason to listen carefully, ask better questions, and evaluate a practitioner the way you'd evaluate any serious clinician: not by whether they recite the same explanation as everyone else, but by whether their reasoning is coherent, their interventions are safe, and their attention to your response is alive.

A PRACTICAL WAY TO HOLD THIS HISTORY (WITHOUT GETTING LOST IN IT)

When patients ask me, "Where did this medicine come from?" they're often asking something more personal: *Is this grounded? Is it reliable? Is it just belief?*

The most honest answer is:

- It came from people paying attention for a very long time.
- It was shaped by the needs of agriculture and governance.
- It was refined by scholar-physicians who wrote clinical arguments, not self-help philosophy.
- It was later standardized into TCM to survive and to scale.
- It still contains multiple voices because human bodies are variable and clinical reality is layered.

If you hold that frame, a lot of confusion dissolves.

You stop demanding that Chinese medicine be either ancient mysticism or modern biomedicine in costume. You stop treating disagreement as proof of fraud. You begin to see the real task: learning how to think clinically in a way that respects complexity without worshiping it.

In the next chapter, we'll move from origins to the central method that ties classical practice together: how Chinese medicine organizes clinical information into patterns—and how those patterns guide decisions in real time.

3

Maps, Not Organs

If you've ever had to describe pain to someone who couldn't feel it —"It's sharp, but also deep… it moves… it's worse when I'm stressed… it's better with heat."—You already know the central problem of medicine: experience doesn't arrive in neat categories.

A clinician's job is to turn lived, messy, subjective reality into something you can act on without betraying it. That requires a map.

In the previous chapters, we've already acknowledged something important: modern anatomy and modern tools are extraordinary, and structural thinking can become a kind of trance when it's the only map in the room. Chinese medicine doesn't compete with anatomy. It offers a different kind of cartography—one that's less about naming parts and more about tracking relationships.

This chapter is about that shift: from organs as objects to physiology as networks; from "where is it?" to "what is it doing, and how is it moving (or failing to move)?" It's about learning to hear classical terms—*Liver, Spleen, Kidney, Heart*—as metaphors for functional systems rather than literal lumps of tissue. And it's about why, clinically, that distinction isn't philosophical. It changes what you notice, what you ignore, and what you try first.

THE BODY UNDERSTOOD THROUGH NETWORKS AND RELATIONSHIPS

When people first encounter Chinese medicine, they often assume it's an older, simpler model—an antique anatomy with different labels. But classical Chinese medicine isn't trying to be anatomy at all. It's trying to be physiology as lived and observed: patterns that recur across many people over a long timescale.

That constraint shaped the entire system.

If you can't look inside, you learn to listen outside. You build a medicine from what the body *does*: how it warms, cools, moistens, dries, moves, stores, transforms, protects, and communicates. You watch what changes with seasons, stress, food, sleep, aging, childbirth, and overwork. You notice how one complaint predicts another—how migraines travel with tight ribs, how insomnia travels with night sweats, how loose stools travel with fatigue and worry.

These are not "mystical correspondences." They're network observations.

In the clinic, network thinking shows up in practical ways:

- A symptom in one place is often driven by a dynamic elsewhere.
- The body doesn't fail one organ at a time; it compensates until it can't.
- Chronic problems tend to be stabilized by feedback loops—patterns that keep recreating themselves.

So the classical project becomes: *What are the stable loops? Where are the leverage points? What relationship is stuck?*

You can do that kind of reasoning with modern physiology too—neuroendocrine loops, inflammatory cascades, autonomic imbalance, motor patterns, pain sensitization. Chinese medicine simply built its own vocabulary for similar kinds of relational thinking, and it built treatment methods that test those relationships directly.

That last part matters. A map is only as good as what it lets you do, and the test is in the clinic.

CHANNELS AS CONDUITS OF MOVEMENT, NOT LINES ON SKIN

Most people encounter the "meridians" as drawings: clean lines on a textbook body, dots with strange names and a numbering system that looks like subway stops. It's understandable to assume channels are literal tubes under the skin—some invisible plumbing that needles "open."

But clinically, that interpretation breaks down quickly.

The classical channel system is better understood as a map of movement and communication through the body. It tracks how certain qualities—heat, cold, tension, sensation, weakness, swelling, numbness—tend to *travel.* It maps where symptoms *refer*, where pain *echoes*, and where dysfunction in one region predicts changes in another.

A channel is a conduit in the same way a watershed is a conduit. You don't need a physical pipe to have a predictable flow.

Here's what this looks like in real treatment.

A patient comes in with pain on the outside of the knee, sharp on stairs. Their MRI shows mild degeneration—nothing dramatic. Physical therapy helps a bit, then plateaus. On palpation, their lateral thigh feels like a taut cable, their hip is restricted, and the side of their neck is also tight and tender in a very specific band. They also mention headaches that wrap around the temple when work gets intense.

If I'm only thinking "knee," I'll live inside the knee. If I'm thinking of channels as movement maps, I'll recognize a common pathway: lateral body tension patterns that link the hip, the iliotibial tract region, the lateral knee, the temple, and the side neck. Needling certain distal points on the lower leg can soften the neck within minutes - but only if this is the reason the neck is tight, and there are many potential reasons. Rechecking the knee after the neck releases isn't magic; it's a test of a relationship.

What moved?

Not a line on the skin. The patient's tone changed. Their neuromuscular holding pattern shifted. Their perception of the knee changed because the larger pattern governing that region changed.

Channels are useful because the body isn't organized by our specialties. It's organized by functional integration: fascia, nerves, vessels, motor patterns, autonomic reflexes, inflammatory signaling, and learned stress responses. Classical clinicians didn't name those structures, but they were tracking the same practical reality: influence travels.

"But are channels real?"

It depends on what you mean by *real.*

If you mean "are they a distinct anatomical structure you can dissect," that's the wrong question. The channel system is closer to a functional overlay: a way of predicting where to look, where to palpate, where to treat, and how a change in one zone will show up in another.

The more honest clinical question is: *Does it improve perception and decision-making? Does it help you test hypotheses with treatment? Does thinking this way get you out of pain??*

Used well, the channel map makes you less literal and more observant. Used poorly, it becomes superstition: a set of lines you follow without listening to the person in front of you. The map is not the terrain.

The channels are about movement—so stagnation matters

Once you think in conduits, you start to notice that many chronic problems have the same flavor: things aren't moving well.

That can mean different things:

- Blood flow and microcirculation
- Lymphatic and interstitial fluid dynamics
- GI motility
- Respiratory excursion and rib mechanics

- Autonomic flexibility (ability to shift gears)
- Emotional processing that loops instead of actually completing.

Classical language often gathers these under the idea of *constraint*, *stagnation*, or *obstruction*—words that can sound abstract until you palpate a body that feels bound up like rope, or you watch someone's symptoms flare every time they try to rest because their system can't downshift.

In those cases, a channel-based approach is not "treating energy." It's choosing interventions that restore change and circulation—mechanical, neurological, vascular, perceptual. The map helps you organize that intention.

ZANG FU AS FUNCTIONAL DOMAINS: TRANSFORMATION AND STORAGE

Now we come to the terms that confuse almost everyone: *Liver, Spleen, Kidney, Heart, Lung*.

We've already touched on the core idea earlier: these names point to systems of function, not the isolated anatomical organ. This chapter is where we go deeper—because the deeper you go, the more you realize the translation problem isn't cosmetic. It can distort clinical reasoning.

In classical physiology, the *Zang* and *Fu* are categories of function.

- **Zang** are associated with the *storage* and regulation of core substances and capacities.
- **Fu** are associated with *transformation, transport, and processing*—more movement, more throughput.

This isn't a perfect match to any modern structure. It's a clinical scaffold: a way to track how the body maintains reserves, processes inputs, distributes resources, and eliminates waste.

Think of it less like "organs" and more like *departments* in an organization. The accounting department might sit in one room, but accounting happens throughout the company. If you think accounting is only in that room, you'll miss what's actually going wrong.

Storage and transformation: a practical lens

Many chronic illnesses can be framed as a mismatch between:

- what the body can **transform** day-to-day (food, stress, sensory load, emotional load, environmental demands)
- and what the body can **store** as stable capacity (sleep quality, hormonal resilience, blood volume, immune tolerance, connective tissue integrity, attentional bandwidth)

Some people are good at throughput but have poor reserves. They can hustle until they crash. Others have reserves but poor movement; they accumulate, bloat, get stuck, and get foggy. Others have neither, and everything feels like too much.

Classical Zang Fu language gives you a structured way to ask: *Is the issue mainly processing? distribution? containment? cooling? warming? storing? letting go?* These are functional questions that guide treatment.

WHY ORGAN NAMES ARE METAPHORS FOR SYSTEMS, NOT ANATOMY

The classical terms were never meant to be read as gross anatomy. The problem is that English makes it almost impossible not to.

If I tell you, "This looks like a Liver pattern," your mind immediately goes to the liver—bilirubin, enzymes, fatty change, hepatitis. That's not irrational. That's the meaning of the word *liver* in modern life.

But in classical usage, "Liver" is shorthand for a set of observed functions: regulation of smooth flow, integration with tendons, certain emotional and sensory patterns, and a particular style of constraint and heat generation under stress. None of that requires pathology in the anatomical liver—though sometimes there may be overlap.

The classical authors weren't ignorant of the physical organs; they simply weren't building a medical system around dissection. Their primary unit of analysis was the function as it appears in the living person.

A clinical example: "Liver" without liver disease

A patient has:

- headaches that worsen with frustration
- tight upper trapezius and jaw clenching
- irregular digestion—alternating constipation and loose stools
- a wiry pulse, red sides of the tongue
- symptoms that worsen before menstruation

A purely structural map might lead you to "migraine management," "TMJ," "IBS," "PMS," each with separate protocols. A classical map sees an integrated pattern: a system that's trying to move and can't, building pressure and heat, then discharging it through the head, neck, gut, and cycle.

Calling this "Liver constraint" (or a related pattern) doesn't mean the person's liver is sick. It means the *regulatory function* that keeps the movement smooth is failing under load.

Treatment, accordingly, isn't aimed at an organ. It's aimed at restoring smooth movement and removing blockages in the appropriate channel (s).

A clinical example: "Spleen" without a spleen problem

Another patient has:

- fatigue after meals
- bloating, loose stools, heaviness in the limbs
- brain fog that worsens with worry and overthinking
- a tendency to bruise easily
- a pale, swollen tongue with teeth marks

This is often called "Spleen Qi deficiency with dampness." If you take the word *" spleen "* literally, you'll think we're discussing an anatomical spleen disorder. We're not. We're describing a functional domain: digestion, transformation, fluid handling, and the kind of cognitive rumination that correlates with it in real bodies.

Again: not mystical. Observational.

Many people with this pattern have perfectly normal imaging and labs. Their problem is functional: motility, absorption, autonomic tone, inflammatory sensitivity, and the metabolic cost of chronic stress. The classical "Spleen" system is a way to integrate those facts into a coherent plan.

"Kidney" and the problem of literal fear

"Kidney" is the most dangerous translation of all, because it can frighten patients.

In classical language, "Kidney" has to do with reserves: growth, development, reproduction, bones, hearing, deep constitutional strength, and the capacity to adapt over time. When someone is exhausted to the marrow— low back weakness, tinnitus, poor recovery, fearfulness, night urination, thinning hair—classical clinicians often speak in Kidney terms.

If a patient hears "Kidney deficiency" and thinks "renal failure," you've created unnecessary fear and confusion. Not because the map is wrong, but because the translation is unskillful.

A good clinician protects the patient from the map's pitfalls. You use the map to guide treatment, not to impose a narrative that terrifies or misleads.

THE DANGER OF LITERAL TRANSLATION WITHOUT CLINICAL CONTEXT

Translation isn't only about words. It's about *what a word makes someone assume.*

Classical Chinese medical terms are compressed. They're more like labels on a file folder than definitions. They assume shared clinical training and a shared set of observations. When you lift those labels into English and present them to modern readers without context, the meaning warps.

A few common distortions:

1) Mistaking metaphor for mechanism

Saying "Wind" doesn't mean air is inside you. It means sudden change, movement, shifting symptoms—tremors, spasms, dizziness, rashes that move, pain that migrates. It's a metaphor for behavior.

When metaphors are taken as literal substances, Chinese medicine becomes easy to mock—and harder to practice well.

2) Mistaking classical categories for biomedical diagnoses

If a patient has "Heart heat," we're not diagnosing myocarditis. We're describing a pattern that might include insomnia, agitation, mouth ulcers, a red tongue tip—often a stress physiology picture.

Likewise, "Phlegm" can refer to much more than mucus: nodules, foggy thinking, heaviness, metabolic congestion, certain types of anxiety. If you insist it must be sputum, you miss the clinical reality the word is pointing toward.

3) Treating words as entities rather than shorthand

In inexperienced hands, a term becomes a thing: "You have dampness." As if "dampness" is a creature living in the body.

In experienced hands, the term stays what it was meant to be:

shorthand for a cluster of signs and tendencies that guide strategy. The difference is enormous.

4) Skipping the step of palpation and direct observation

One reason literal translation proliferates is that words are easier than bodies. You can memorize terms and argue about them without touching a patient.

But classical medicine is tactile and observational. It's built around pulse, abdomen, channels, temperature, voice, smell, eyes, and the way symptoms change under pressure, heat, breath, emotion, and treatment.

Without that clinical context, the map becomes a belief system. With it, it becomes a tool.

HOW MAPS GUIDE PERCEPTION RATHER THAN REPLACE REALITY

A good map doesn't tell you what's there. It tells you what to look for and how to relate what you find.

If you've ever used a topographical map while hiking, you know the feeling: the terrain is real, but the map trains your eyes. You start noticing ridgelines, drainage, slopes, saddles. You see patterns in the land you would have missed.

Chinese medicine is like that. It trains perception toward certain relationships:

- surface and interior
- movement and storage
- excess and deficiency
- heat and cold
- dryness and dampness
- constraint and release
- ascending and descending
- harmonizing versus purging, tonifying versus dispersing

None of these are "things" you can hold. They're ways the living system behaves.

The danger isn't that these categories are false. The danger is that we forget they are *categories* and begin treating them as reality itself.

The map is not the patient

In clinic, the patient will violate your model regularly.

Someone will have all the textbook signs of "cold" and still crave cold drinks. Someone will have a red tongue and still respond to warming herbs. Someone will have a "perfect" pulse and look exhausted. Someone's pain will break every rule.

If your map can't tolerate those moments, it becomes a prison. If it can, it becomes what it was meant to be: a guide, not a replacement for attention.

One of the most practical skills in classical work is learning when to lean on the map and when to set it down and re-contact the person.

WHY MULTIPLE MAPS CAN COEXIST WITHOUT CONTRADICTION

A patient can be described accurately in multiple languages at once.

Take a person with chronic reflux and anxiety:

- A gastroenterologist might see LES tone issues, hypersensitivity, delayed gastric emptying, and stress-mediated symptom amplification.
- A nervous system lens might see sympathetic dominance, vagal underactivity, and interoceptive threat loops.
- A musculoskeletal lens might see a tight diaphragm, rib flare, forward head posture, and breathing patterns that perpetuate thoracic tension.
- A Chinese medicine lens might see rebellious Stomach

Qi, constraint in the regulatory system, and heat or phlegm patterns depending on the presentation.

These are not mutually exclusive. They are maps that highlight different relationships.

Contradiction only appears if you demand that one map be the *territory*. If you insist that "real" means "visible under a microscope," you'll discard functional phenomena that are clinically obvious. If you insist that classical categories are literal substances, you'll reject anatomy and physiology that are clearly true.

A mature clinician can move between maps without ideological drama.

Sometimes you need the structural map first. If someone has red flags—weight loss, bleeding, neurologic deficits—you don't soothe yourself with pattern language. You refer out. You image. You rule out what must be ruled out.

Sometimes the structural map is necessary but insufficient. Imaging can be normal, and suffering can be severe. Labs can be "fine" while the person can't sleep, digest, or regulate mood. In those cases, functional maps become clinically necessary.

The coexistence of maps isn't a compromise. It's reality. The body is too complex for one vocabulary.

FUNCTIONAL HEURISTICS VERSUS OBJECTIVE FACTS

This is where people get uneasy. They want to know: *Is Chinese medicine true?*

It depends on what kind of truth you're asking for.

If you want objective facts in the way anatomy offers them—structures you can display—classical Chinese medicine isn't that kind of system. It's not claiming that "Liver Qi" is a measurable fluid.

What it offers are **functional heuristics**: reliable, field-tested ways of organizing complex information so you can act.

A heuristic is not a guess. It's a shortcut built from experience. In medicine, heuristics can be lifesaving—or misleading—depending on how intelligently they're applied.

The classical heuristics are not arbitrary. They're built from:

- repeated clinical observation
- pattern clustering
- long-term tracking of outcomes
- an insistence on correlation across multiple signs (not single symptoms)
- and, crucially, the ability to test a hypothesis by treating it

In other words, they are pragmatic.

The honesty required by heuristics

A heuristic requires humility because it's always provisional. You don't get to say, "This is the diagnosis, therefore reality must conform." You say, "This is the current working pattern; let's see if the body agrees."

A good classical clinician is constantly asking:

- If I treat this relationship, does the system shift?
- If it shifts, does it shift in a stable way?
- If it doesn't, what did I misunderstand?
- What did I overvalue? What did I ignore?

This is not mystical. It's iterative reasoning in a complex system.

Why objective facts still matter

Functional thinking doesn't replace objective evaluation. It lives alongside it.

If a patient has anemia, you don't call it "Blood deficiency" and move on. You ask why. You check iron studies. You consider bleeding, absorption, inflammation. You integrate maps.

If a patient has hypothyroidism, you don't pretend that

needles alone will rebuild a thyroid. But you might still treat the fatigue, sleep, digestion, mood, and pain patterns that persist even when TSH normalizes—because the person is more than a lab value.

A clinician who can't respect objective facts becomes untrustworthy. A clinician who can't work with function becomes limited.

MAP VERSUS TERRITORY: THE QUESTION OF CLINICAL UTILITY

"Map versus territory" is one of those phrases that can become a slogan. In clinic, it's more concrete.

The territory is the living person: - their sleep that breaks at 3 a.m. - their neck that tightens after emails - their digestion that collapses under deadlines - their grief that never metabolizes - their pain that moves when they breathe - their period that changes when they travel - their pulse today, not in a book.

The map is what helps you choose: - where to needle - what to warm or cool - what to move or tonify - what to drain or harmonize - what to prioritize this week - what to leave alone until the system is ready.

A map is good if it helps you do those things with fewer wrong turns.

Clinical utility is not the same as scientific explanation

A common confusion is to demand that a map explain *why* something works at the mechanistic level before you allow it to be useful.

Mechanisms matter. But medicine has always used interventions before fully understanding them. Aspirin relieved pain before prostaglandins were named. Handwashing reduced mortality before germ theory was mature. Physical therapy works even when we can't predict exactly which cue will unlock a person's movement pattern.

The classical maps are similar. They are not excuses to avoid science; they are ways to operate skillfully in complexity while science continues to refine the underlying mechanisms.

The practical measure remains: can this map reliably guide effective decisions?

MAPS AS LENSES FOR SEEING DIFFERENT RELATIONSHIPS

One of the most liberating things about classical Chinese medicine —when taught well—is that it permits multiple lenses without forcing them into one hierarchy.

Different lenses reveal different relationships.

The channel lens: where the body speaks through pathways

This lens is especially good for:

- pain patterns
- referred symptoms
- surface-to-interior relationships
- quick clinical testing (needle a distal point, reassess range of motion or tenderness)
- understanding why symptoms travel together along recognizable routes

It tends to excel when the complaint is dynamic: moving pain, episodic flares, "it comes and goes," symptoms triggered by posture or stress.

The Zang Fu lens: how systems allocate resources over time

This lens is especially good for:

- chronic fatigue and burnout patterns

- digestive and fluid regulation issues
- sleep and emotional regulation
- menstrual and fertility patterns
- aging, recovery, and constitutional strength

It shines when you need to build a medium- to long-term strategy: not just symptom suppression, but functional rebuilding.

The six conformations / external-internal lens (another map)

Even without formally naming it, many classical clinicians use a lens that tracks how the body relates to an external or internal "pathogen" (sometimes that pathogen is literal—an infection; sometimes it's metaphorical—an inflammatory state, a lingering stress imprint). This lens can be remarkably useful in:

- chronic post-viral pictures
- alternating chills and feverish sensations
- patterns that shift from one stage to another
- cases where the body feels like it's "fighting something" but can't finish

Again, it's not about believing in an ephemeral "pathogen." It's about recognizing staged physiological struggles.

The Five Phase lens: tendency, temperament, and system style

This lens is often misused as personality typing. Used well, it's subtler: it helps you see *style*—how a person tends to react, where they compensate, what they overuse, what they avoid, what kind of imbalance they produce under load.

In practice, it can help with:

- why two patients with "the same diagnosis" need different treatment pacing
- how emotion and physiology entangle for this particular person
- where compliance will break down (not from laziness, but from a mismatch)

Not every case requires this lens. But when it fits, it can prevent you from treating the pattern while ignoring the person.

A QUIET BUT IMPORTANT WARNING: WHEN THE MAP BECOMES A COSTUME

There's a version of Chinese medicine that performs its maps rather than uses them.

It sounds confident. It uses the terms fluently. It gives the patient an identity—"You are a damp-heat constitution"—and then treats that identity for months.

Sometimes it helps anyway, because they begin directionally correct. But then it stalls, because the practitioner stopped thinking. And the patient changed, which was the goal all along.

The classical tradition, at its best, is not interested in costume. It's interested in *contact*: contact with physiology as it is today, in this person, under these constraints.

A map should make you more responsive, not more rigid.

If the patient changes, the map must change. If the treatment doesn't shift the system, you don't defend the map—you revisit your reading of the territory.

That's not a critique of Chinese medicine. It's a defense of it.

WHAT THIS MEANS FOR YOU (PATIENT OR PRACTITIONER)

If you're a patient, here's the simplest translation:

- When your practitioner says "Liver," they may be talking about a functional pattern, not your anatomical liver.
- When they needle a point far from your complaint, they may be treating a pathway relationship, not "sending energy" across the body in a magical way.
- When they ask about sleep, stool, temperature, mood, and appetite—even if you came in for pain—they may be looking for the network that keeps recreating the pain.

You're allowed to ask: "Do you mean the actual organ?" A good clinician will welcome that question and answer in plain language.

If you're a practitioner or student, the invitation is more demanding:

- Learn the maps, but don't worship them.
- Translate classical terms into functional meaning without flattening them into modern diagnoses.
- Keep returning to palpation, observation, and outcome.
- Treat each map as a lens that reveals relationships—and be willing to switch lenses when the picture doesn't resolve.

A map earns its place by making you more effective and more humane: fewer dead ends, less blame on the patient, more coherent strategy.

CLOSING: WHY THIS CHAPTER MATTERS BEFORE WE GO FURTHER

We can't build clinical skill on a misunderstanding.

If you think Chinese medicine is an alternative anatomy, you'll either dismiss it or practice it mechanically. If you think it's pure symbolism, you'll drift into vagueness. If you recognize it as a set of functional maps—imperfect, evolving, field-tested—you can use it the way it was intended: as a disciplined art of pattern recognition and strategic intervention.

In the next chapters, we'll start working more explicitly with these maps in practice: how information is gathered, how patterns are prioritized, and how treatment becomes a form of inquiry—an ongoing conversation with the body rather than a single pronouncement.

The goal isn't to replace reality with a map.

It's to choose a map that helps you find your way through the territory—especially when the territory is complicated, chronic, and human.

4

Pattern Recognition as a Medical Skill

Most people come to a clinic with a symptom in hand like a receipt.

"My knee hurts."

"I can't sleep."

"My digestion is a mess."

"I'm anxious all the time."

Symptoms are honest. They are also incomplete. They're what the body is willing—or forced—to say out loud. They are surface information: the audible alarm, the dashboard light, the smoke that finally made it out from under the door.

And this is where the trouble starts.

Because if you treat symptoms as *the problem*, you will naturally reach for symptom-shaped solutions: a stronger anti-inflammatory, a better brace, a different pillow, a more restrictive diet, a new supplement, another round of imaging, another specialist. Sometimes that works. Sometimes it doesn't. Sometimes it works briefly, and then the body finds a new way to complain.

What Chinese medicine asks—quietly but insistently—is something slightly different: not "What is the symptom?" but "What kind of body produces this symptom, under these conditions, in this way?" The symptom matters. But it matters as evidence of a deeper organization.

That deeper organization is what we call a *pattern*.

You've already met this idea in earlier chapters: pattern recognition isn't mystical, and it isn't a rejection of modern diagnosis. It's a different level of clinical reasoning—one that tries to find the single coherent functional picture that could plausibly generate the whole cluster at once.

In this chapter, we'll go deeper. Not into more terminology, but into the skill itself: how patterns unify disparate signs, why a complaint like knee pain can belong to digestion or emotion or constitution, why "diagnosis" in this medicine is synthetic rather than categorical, and why treatment follows perception—not labels.

SYMPTOMS ARE SURFACE INFORMATION

A symptom is the part of a story that rises above the waterline.

Think about how people describe a problem when they first sit down:

- "It started in my knee."
- "It's mostly my stomach."
- "It's my hormones."
- "It's my stress."

None of those statements are wrong. They're just incomplete. They are the chapter titles, not the plot.

In the clinic, symptoms are often the *loudest* signal, not the *most informative* one. The loudest signal is what got the person to act. But bodies don't always shout from the source. They shout from the place that can shout.

A simple example from everyday life: if you're sleep-deprived, you might notice irritability first—not because the irritability is the "cause," but because it's the part that impacts your relationships. If you're overloaded at work, you might notice neck tension first—not because your trapezius is the root of your life, but because the body stores certain kinds of strain in certain places.

In medicine, we can confuse the loudest symptom for the primary problem. That confusion is reinforced by how modern care is organized: symptoms are triaged into categories, matched to specialists and treated within those categories. Knee goes to orthopedics. Digestion goes to gastroenterology. Anxiety goes to psychiatry. Skin goes to dermatology.

This division has real strengths. It's how we get precision procedures, targeted drugs, and life-saving interventions. But it also has a cost: it trains us to think of the body as separable objects and isolated failures.

Chinese medicine starts from a different habit of mind: the body as an interdependent function, where a disturbance in one area changes the conditions in another. Symptoms, in that frame, are not the unit of truth. They are the unit of complaint.

So the first clinical task is not to argue with the symptom—"No, your knee pain is actually your digestion"—but to place it in context. What else is happening? What patterns of timing, triggers, and relief surround it? What other systems changed around the same time? What did the body lose the ability to do smoothly?

If symptoms are surface information, then patterns are the underlying organization that makes those symptoms predictable.

PATTERNS ARE UNDERLYING ORGANIZATION

A pattern is not a diagnosis in the usual categorical sense. It is a description of how the person's physiology is currently organizing itself.

That sounds abstract until you feel it clinically.

A pattern has a texture. It has momentum. It has "rules." When you see enough of them, you start to recognize how the body behaves under certain internal conditions—like weather systems. You can't point to one cloud and say, "That cloud caused the storm." But you can recognize a pressure system moving through.

Patterns are not metaphors we use because we don't know the "real" cause. They're functional descriptions: how regulation is failing, compensating, rerouting, or stalling.

A few examples of the kinds of organizing principles that matter clinically:

- **Distribution:** Is the problem rising upward (headaches, insomnia, agitation), sinking downward (diarrhea, heaviness, fatigue), or trapped in the middle (bloating, tight chest, alternating constipation and loose stool)?
- **Quality of movement:** Is the system constrained and stuck, or leaking and collapsing, or flaring and overactive?
- **Relationship between systems:** Is digestion failing to transform and distribute? Is respiration failing to descend? Is circulation failing to warm and nourish? Is the body overreacting to normal input?
- **Time:** Does it worsen at night, after eating, before menstruation, with exertion, with rest, with emotional stress, with weather changes?
- **Compensation:** What is the body doing to cope? Some patterns look like "excess" until you realize the excess is a last-ditch compensation for deficiency.

These aren't just poetic categories. They guide palpation, questioning, and treatment selection. They tell you what to look for next. A good pattern doesn't merely summarize; it predicts. If you think you see a certain pattern, you should be able to ask the next question and get a confirming answer far more often than chance would allow.

That is what makes pattern recognition a medical skill rather than a storytelling exercise. It is testable, revisable, and anchored in physiology—not physiology as a list of organs, but as coordinated function.

DIAGNOSIS AS SYNTHETIC RATHER THAN CATEGORICAL

Most biomedical diagnoses are categorical. You either meet the criteria or you don't. Categories matter: they determine prognosis, rule out dangerous conditions, and guide standardized treatment.

But categories can also become a trap when they are treated as if they *explain* a person rather than *classify* a condition.

Chinese medicine diagnosis—at least when practiced with care—is synthetic. It's not trying to decide which box you belong in. It's trying to assemble a coherent picture from multiple streams of evidence:

- what you feel,
- what we observe,
- what the pulse and abdomen and tissue tone suggest,
- what your sleep and digestion and temperature regulation are doing,
- what your history and constitution have set up,
- what your emotions do to your body, and what your body does to your emotions.

The synthesis is the diagnosis.

This is why the questions can feel oddly broad when you came in for something specific. Someone walks in with knee pain, and I ask about stool quality, urination, sweating, sleep timing, appetite, cold hands, menstrual history, afternoon fatigue, nightmares, irritability, thirst, and whether the pain changes with weather.

It's not because I think everything is everything. It's because a knee is not a closed ecosystem.

A categorical diagnosis often points to a named entity: osteoarthritis, meniscus tear or patellofemoral syndrome. Those categories are real and useful. But they don't automatically tell you why *this* person is experiencing it *now*, why it flares under certain conditions, why recovery stalls, or why the pain spreads, migrates, or changes character.

A synthetic diagnosis tries to answer those questions. It's a map of the current terrain rather than a label on the file.

There's another important consequence: in a synthetic system, multiple patterns can coexist. People rarely present as a single clean pattern. They are layered: a constitution underneath, a life lived on top, an acute insult over that, and compensations everywhere.

A good practitioner is not hunting for the one perfect term. They're trying to understand which layer is driving the presentation today—and which lever will shift the whole system with the least force.

UNIFYING DISPARATE SIGNS

One of the quiet miracles of good pattern recognition is the moment disparate signs stop being "multiple problems" and start being one picture.

A patient might list these as separate issues:

- headaches,
- jaw tension,
- irritable bowel,
- PMS,
- waking at 3 a.m.,
- tight shoulders,
- sighing,
- a sense of being "wired but tired."

In a symptom-based frame, that is a long checklist and a long plan: magnesium for headaches, mouth guard for jaw, probiotics for gut, something for sleep, maybe an SSRI for mood, stretching for shoulders.

In a pattern-based frame, those features might unify around a constrained regulatory dynamic: the system is not moving and distributing smoothly. Pressure builds. Sleep becomes light and interrupted. Digestion becomes reactive. Pain shows up in tendons and connective tissue. Mood becomes irritable, not because the person is "emotionally dysregulated" in a moral sense, but because their physiology is living with chronic internal friction.

Once the pattern coheres, treatment becomes more elegant. Not easier—humans aren't easy—but more coherent. You're not chasing symptoms across the body like a person trying to plug leaks in a roof during a storm. You're addressing the pressure system.

This unification is not theoretical. It is experienced by the patient as relief that makes sense.

They'll say things like:

"I didn't realize my sleep and digestion were connected."

"My knee still aches sometimes, but I feel like myself again."

"It's not just one symptom getting better. It's like my whole baseline changed."

That's a signal you're working at the level of organization rather than the level of isolated complaints.

And it's also a form of respect. When a patient has been told for years that their symptoms are unrelated—or worse, that they're exaggerating because no single test explains the whole list—pattern recognition offers another possibility: that the body is consistent, even when the medical system can't easily categorize it.

WHY KNEE PAIN CAN BE DIGESTIVE, EMOTIONAL, OR CONSTITUTIONAL

This is the part that tends to sound like overreach until you've seen it enough times.

How could knee pain have anything to do with digestion? Or grief? Or a person's constitution?

The answer is not that "everything causes everything." The answer is that pain is a language, and the knee is a common place where several systemic dynamics can become legible.

Let's stay grounded. There are local reasons knees hurt: injury, degeneration, biomechanics, inflammation, meniscal pathology, referred pain from the hip or back. If there is swelling, instability, locking, trauma, fever, or unexplained weight loss—those are not philosophical discussions. Those are medical priorities.

But once serious pathology is ruled out, we often face a different question: why does pain persist? Why does it fluctuate with stress, sleep, food, weather, and fatigue? Why does physical therapy help but not "stick?" Why do some people have terrible imaging and little pain, while others have mild imaging changes and disabling pain?

Pattern recognition gives you additional angles.

1) The digestive connection: nourishment, dampness, and tissue quality

In Chinese medicine, digestion isn't just about breaking down food. It's about transforming input into usable fuel and distributing it—like an internal supply chain.

When that system is weak or burdened, you can see downstream effects in the musculoskeletal system:

- chronic heaviness in the limbs,
- a sense of swelling without obvious swelling,
- slow recovery after exertion,
- tendons and connective tissue that feel undernourished or easily irritated,
- pain that worsens with humidity or after rich foods,
- loose stool, bloating, fatigue after meals.

Through a modern lens, you could interpret this as multiple plausible mechanisms: systemic inflammation, altered microbiome signaling, nutrient absorption issues, glycemic swings, immune activation, changes in connective tissue hydration, and even behavioral patterns around energy and movement.

But you don't have to reduce it to a single mechanism to treat it intelligently. Clinically, you can watch the pattern: when digestion improves, the heaviness lifts; when heaviness lifts, the knee stops feeling like it's carrying a sandbag.

I've had patients with chronic knee pain whose turning point was not a new knee exercise but a treatment plan that stabilized appetite, stool, and post-meal fatigue. The knee didn't "come from" the gut in a simplistic causal chain. The knee was one of the places where a global failure of transformation and distribution became apparent under load.

2) The emotional connection: constraint, tension, and the body's bracing patterns

Emotion is not an add-on to physiology. It is physiology. Not in the sense that "it's all in your head," but in the sense that emotional states change breathing, circulation, muscle tone, digestion, and sleep architecture.

Certain emotional states—especially chronic frustration, grief held in the chest, sustained worry—create predictable changes in how the body moves energy and blood. People brace. Their ribs become less mobile. Their diaphragm gets less forgiving. Their shoulders sit closer to their ears. Their jaw clenches. Their gait changes subtly.

The knee is not immune to this. Chronic bracing changes load patterns through the pelvis and leg. Constraint in the trunk changes how force is transmitted through the hip and knee. This is biomechanics, but it's also neurology and circulation.

In the classical frame, constraint tends to create pressure. Pressure tends to seek outlets. If the outlet is muscular tension, you see tight bands and trigger points. If the outlet is heat, you see agitation and insomnia. If the outlet is digestive reactivity, you see alternating bowel patterns. If the outlet is the joints, you see pain that flares with stress and eases when life softens.

A clinical clue here is variability: knee pain that predictably worsens after emotional conflict, deadline pressure, or periods of suppressed anger—especially when imaging doesn't fully account for severity.

This doesn't mean the pain is "psychological." It means the system is responding to stress through the musculoskeletal channel. Treatment might include points that reduce constraint and restore downward movement, but it also includes pragmatic counseling: changing training intensity, sleep timing, work posture, and learning what emotional compression feels like in the body before it becomes pain.

3) The constitutional connection: resilience, aging, and the deep supply lines

Some knee pain is not primarily due to digestion or emotion. It's constitutional: the baseline resources that maintain joints, bones, and recovery capacity.

Classically, knees are closely tied to deep reserves—what Chinese medicine often frames through the Kidney system (again, not the anatomical organ, but a functional network associated with growth, development, bone, marrow, and long-term resilience).

Constitutional patterns show up as:

- slow healing,
- low back weakness accompanying knee issues,
- fatigue that is deeper than sleep can fix,
- cold intolerance or a sense of diminished fire,
- tinnitus, hair changes, or urinary frequency,
- fearfulness or a loss of willpower that feels physiological, not psychological,
- pain that worsens with overwork and improves with rest and warmth.

This is common after long periods of depletion: years of parenting without sleep, chronic illness, overtraining, grief, burnout, or simply aging. The knee becomes a messenger: "We do not have the surplus for this load anymore."

In those cases, if you treat only the knee locally—needling around the joint, topical herbs, strengthening—you may get partial relief. But lasting improvement usually requires working on the deeper supply lines: warming and supporting the system, improving restorative sleep, pacing exertion, rebuilding capacity over months rather than weeks.

The reason this matters is that it changes the strategy. You don't tell a constitutionally depleted person to "push through" rehab the same way you would a robust 25-year-old athlete. The pattern tells you what kind of effort the body can metabolize.

4) The "mixed pattern" reality: why it's rarely just one thing

Most real knee pain cases are mixed.

A person might have mild degenerative change (structural), plus digestive heaviness (systemic), plus stress-related constraint (regulatory), plus constitutional depletion (recovery deficit). Any one of these might be manageable. Together, they create persistent pain.

Pattern recognition lets you prioritize without oversimplifying. On one visit, the key might be to reduce swelling and pain. On another, the key might be to improve sleep and digestion. On another, it might be to rebuild deep reserves.

When you work this way, the knee becomes less of a mystery. Not because you found "the cause," but because you found the organization that makes the pain behave the way it does.

THE DIFFERENCE BETWEEN NAMING A PATTERN AND UNDERSTANDING IT

This is where a lot of Chinese medicine goes wrong—especially when it's taught as vocabulary.

Students learn lists: Liver Qi stagnation. Spleen Qi deficiency. Damp-heat. Blood stasis. Kidney Yang deficiency. And then they try to match a patient to the nearest phrase.

The phrase becomes a substitute for understanding.

Naming a pattern is nothing. A good name can carry a lot of information, just as "pneumonia" does. But in Chinese medicine, pattern names are compressions. They are shorthand for a relationship.

If you stop at the name, you can miss the living reality:

- Two people can both be called "Spleen Qi deficient" and need very different treatments because one is cold and collapsing, while the other is damp and congested.
- Two people can both be called "Blood stasis," and one needs gentle movement and warming, while the other needs clearing heat and cooling the blood.
- Two people can both be called "Liver Qi stagnation," and one is constrained from grief while the other is constrained from overwork, and their bodies will respond differently.

Understanding a pattern means understanding:

1. **What is the primary dysfunction?** (movement, transformation, containment, warming, cooling, ascent/descent)

2. **What is driving it?** (diet, overthinking, trauma, overtraining, chronic infection, aging, medications, environment)

3. **What is compensating for what?** (Is the "excess" actually a compensatory response?)

4. **What is the direction of change?** (Is the person worsening, stabilizing, or recovering?)

5. **What is the most efficient lever right now?** (What intervention shifts multiple symptoms at once without strain?)

A pattern name can be correct and still clinically useless if it doesn't lead to effective decisions. Conversely, a practitioner might not articulate the perfect classical phrase but still treat brilliantly because they perceive the dynamics accurately.

In other words, the goal is not to become fluent in pattern names. The goal is to become fluent in physiology as a relationship.

This is why classical training emphasizes palpation, pulse, abdomen, temperature, tissue tone, and the patient's narrative—not as separate data points, but as ways of sensing the same underlying organization from different angles.

The body is telling one story. Pattern recognition is the skill of hearing it.

DIAGNOSIS WITHOUT CERTAINTY THEATER

There's a temptation—especially with intelligent patients and conscientious practitioners—to perform certainty.

Patients want answers. Practitioners want to be helpful. "Here's your diagnosis." "Here's what's wrong." "Here's the root."

But chronic, complex presentations rarely grant that kind of clean resolution. If we pretend they do, we end up defending our label instead of updating our understanding.

Pattern recognition, when practiced honestly, includes humility as a technique.

You form a working model. You test it through careful treatment and observation. You watch what shifts and what doesn't. You revise.

This is not a weakness of Chinese medicine. It's one of its strengths: it is designed to be iterative. You don't need to be omniscient at the first visit. You need to be perceptive, methodical, and responsive.

A good pattern diagnosis feels like this:

- It explains more than it ignores.
- It predicts what else might be true.
- It suggests a treatment strategy that is coherent.
- It changes as the patient changes.

If your pattern never changes across months of treatment,

something is off. Either the treatment isn't working, or the practitioner is clinging to an early story because it feels safer than uncertainty.

Real bodies don't reward that kind of rigidity.

TREATMENT FOLLOWS PERCEPTION, NOT LABELS

This may be the most practical point in the entire chapter.

In Chinese medicine, treatment is not chosen because a label was assigned. Treatment is chosen because a *dynamic* was perceived.

Two patients can walk in with the same biomedical diagnosis—say, osteoarthritis of the knee—and receive very different treatments because their patterns differ:

- One has cold, weakness, and deep fatigue: you warm, support, and strengthen the system while gently moving local stagnation.
- Another has swelling, heaviness, sticky digestion, and heat signs: you transform dampness, clear heat, and open pathways.
- Another has stress-linked flares, sighing, chest tightness, and insomnia: you course constraint, settle agitation, and restore smooth regulation.
- Another has sharp fixed pain with a history of injury: you focus more strongly on moving blood, resolving stasis, and restoring tissue function.

Conversely, two patients with different biomedical diagnoses might receive similar treatments because the pattern is similar.

This is one reason Chinese medicine can look confusing from the outside. It doesn't align neatly with disease categories. It aligns with functional states.

When treatment follows perception rather than labels, you also avoid one of the most common clinical traps: treating the pattern name instead of the person.

A pattern name can seduce you into a formula. "This is damp-heat; I will clear damp-heat." But what if clearing damp-heat is too harsh for this person's constitution? What if the damp-heat is secondary to constraint? What if the "heat" is actually deficiency heat from depletion? What if the dampness is from medications? What if the patient is postpartum and needs nourishment first?

Perception keeps you honest. Labels make you lazy.

This doesn't mean you reinvent treatment every time or ignore tradition. Classical medicine has a deep lineage of strategies precisely because practitioners observed patterns over centuries. But the tradition is not a set of rigid recipes. It is a library of tested responses to recognizable dynamics.

A good clinician uses that library the way a musician uses scales: not to impress, but to make something coherent in real time.

A CLINICAL WALKTHROUGH: FROM COMPLAINT TO PATTERN

Let's make this concrete. Imagine a patient comes in with knee pain.

They tell you:

- Pain is worse when going downstairs.
- It's better with warmth.
- It flares before the period.
- They're bloated after meals and crave sweets.
- They have loose stools in the morning.
- They're exhausted in the afternoon.
- They feel puffy when it rains.
- They sleep lightly and wake early, mind busy.

If you treat only the knee, you might needle local points, prescribe anti-inflammatory herbs, and give strengthening exercises. It might help, but the pattern suggests something broader: a system that struggles with transformation (digestive weakness), accumulates heaviness (dampness), and becomes more constrained cyclically (premenstrual worsening).

Now imagine a different knee pain patient:

- Pain is sharp and fixed, in one spot.
- History of an old injury.
- Pain worsens at night.
- The knee feels cold and stiff in the morning.
- They have low back weakness and frequent urination.
- They're sleeping but not restoring.
- They've been burned out for years.

Same symptom: knee pain. Different organization: deeper depletion with local stagnation from old trauma.

And a third:

- Knee pain migrates—sometimes medial, sometimes lateral.
- It flares after arguments or intense work deadlines.
- They have headaches, jaw clenching, and rib-side tightness.
- Digestion alternates—constipation then loose stool.
- Sleep is disrupted, especially waking between 1 and 3 a.m.

Here, the pattern is dominated by constraint and dysregulation of movement. The knee is a recipient of systemic tension.

These aren't contrived. They're common. And they illustrate the central point: the symptom does not tell you the treatment. The pattern does.

WHAT PATTERN RECOGNITION GIVES PATIENTS (AND WHY IT MATTERS)

If you're a patient reading this, you might be thinking: "Fine, but what does this do for me?"

When done well, pattern recognition offers three things many people are starving for:

1) Coherence without oversimplification

You don't have to choose between "everything is unrelated" and "everything is caused by one magic root." Patterns allow a coherent story that can hold multiple truths.

2) A way to track progress that isn't binary

Chronic healing is rarely a straight line. Pattern-based care gives you intermediate markers: sleep depth, stool quality, temperature regulation, mood steadiness, and recovery after exertion. Those changes matter even before the primary symptom fully resolves.

3) A treatment plan that adapts

If your body changes, the treatment changes. If stress increases, we adjust. If digestion stabilizes, we shift focus. If the pain localizes, we treat it differently. This is not an inconsistency; it's responsiveness.

And it can be deeply relieving to have a practitioner who is not trying to force you into a diagnostic box, but is instead trying to understand the logic your body is following—even if you don't like the outcome of that logic.

THE ETHICAL EDGE OF PATTERN RECOGNITION

There is also an ethical dimension to this skill.

When we reduce people to symptoms or categories, we subtly imply that what doesn't fit is irrelevant—or imaginary. Pattern recognition, at its best, refuses that dismissal. It insists that the body is lawful, even when the law isn't obvious yet.

That doesn't mean every symptom will be explained neatly. Some cases remain complex. Some remain partially mysterious. But the stance is different: we keep looking for coherence, and we keep testing our understanding through results.

This is one reason I still value the classical method even in a world with extraordinary imaging and lab testing. Those tools can tell you what tissue looks like. Pattern recognition can tell you how the person is functioning—and why the same tissue finding can mean different things in different bodies.

Both matter. They answer different questions.

CLOSING: LEARNING TO SEE THE WHOLE PICTURE

A symptom is a doorway. Pattern recognition is what happens when you walk through it instead of decorating the door.

It's a clinical skill built from attention: attention to timing, triggers, relief, sensation quality, emotional tone, digestion, sleep, temperature, constitution, and the way the pulse and tissues tell the same story in another language.

It asks you to trade the comfort of a single cause for the clarity of a coherent pattern. Not because certainty is bad, but because premature certainty is expensive. It costs patients time, money, hope, and sometimes years of chasing the wrong target.

In the next chapter, we'll get more specific about how this skill is trained in practice—how a practitioner learns to gather information without getting lost in it, how palpation becomes a way of thinking, and how treatment itself becomes part of the diagnostic process.

For now, keep one idea close: in Chinese medicine, the label is not the medicine. Perception is the medicine. Treatment follows what you can actually see.

5

The Language of the Living Body

People often ask about pulse and tongue diagnosis the way they ask about lie detectors—*Do they really work?* As if the question is whether a technique is "real," rather than whether a clinician can learn to perceive what the body is already expressing.

That's an understandable question. In a medical culture trained to trust numbers, images, and named diseases, pulse and tongue can sound like relics—ceremonial, symbolic, maybe comforting, maybe suspicious. But in clinic, these methods don't function as symbols. They function as **interfaces**—ways of meeting physiology in motion.

And if you've been reading along, you already know the larger frame: this medicine is not primarily about objects; it's about **relationships**—how systems coordinate, how symptoms speak for networks, how a body tries to regulate itself under imperfect conditions. Pulse and tongue are two of the oldest ways to listen to that regulation without interrupting it.

Not because the ancients were mystical, but because they were attentive. They didn't have imaging. They had something else: long observation, repeated contact, and a clinical culture that treated perception as a skill you can refine—like music, carpentry, or cooking. Not a belief. A craft.

The Pulse as a Dialogue

In most modern settings, "pulse" means a number. Maybe rhythm. Maybe it's strong or weak. We check it quickly and move on, because the pulse is mainly used as a warning light: too fast, too slow, irregular, thready in shock.

In classical practice, the pulse is not a warning light. It's a **conversation**.

Not in a romantic sense. In a technical sense. When your fingers rest on the radial artery, you're not just detecting pressure waves. You're meeting the ongoing negotiation between:

- the heart's propulsion
- the vessels' tone and compliance
- the volume and viscosity of blood and fluids
- autonomic balance and stress chemistry
- temperature regulation
- the body's current strategy: conserve, spend, fight, rest, repair

That's already a lot. And it gets more interesting when you remember that symptoms are rarely isolated. The pulse can show you whether the symptoms are the main event—or the smoke from a deeper fire.

A patient tells you, "I'm exhausted, but wired at night." Another tells you, "My digestion is off, and my mood is flat." A third says, "My periods are clotty and painful." Their stories may overlap.

Their diagnoses in a conventional system might overlap too: insomnia, IBS, dysmenorrhea. But their pulses often do not overlap.

Because the pulse is not a category. It's a *state.*

And that's why we call it a dialogue. When you palpate the pulse in this tradition, you are asking a series of questions with your hands:

- Is the circulation moving freely, or pushing through resistance?
- Is the body distributing resources, or hoarding them?
- Are fluids adequate, or being consumed faster than they can be replenished?
- Is the system resilient, or lacking adaptive capacity??
- Is the person running on reserve or on stress?

The body answers in a language that is tactile, rhythmic, and layered. You don't get "yes" or "no." You get texture.

Beyond Rate and Rhythm: What the Fingers Actually Perceive

It's worth being specific here, because vague language is where pulse diagnosis gets caricatured.

A trained palpation is not one impression. It is several observations gathered consistently. Different lineages emphasize different maps, but the core idea remains stable: you assess the pulse at multiple positions and depths and pay attention to qualities that reflect more than just hemodynamics.

Some of what's perceived includes:

- **Depth**: Does the pulse present itself strongly at the surface, deeper down, or throughout? A surface-dominant pulse can correlate with acute, exterior processes—think of the body mobilizing resources to its boundaries. A deep-dominant pulse often shows internal load, internal cold, internal constraint, or simply a system that is not broadcasting outward.

- **Width and shape**: Is it fine like a thread, broad like a rope, rounded like a bead, sharp like a taut string? These aren't poetic flourishes; they're tactile phenomena that correlate with fluid status, tension, and the manner in which force is being transmitted.
- **Strength and root**: Does it have substance when you press down, or does it collapse? Does it feel like it rises to meet your finger, or like it retreats? This is one place where you can sense the difference between "energetic" and "resourced." Many people appear to have good energy, but are largely running on stress. This is reflected in the pulse's rootedness.
- **Tension and elasticity**: Is the vessel compliant or stiff? Is the pulse relaxed, tight, wiry, urgent? This can mirror a sympathetic tone, pain patterns, chest or diaphragmatic constraint or long-standing stress physiology.
- **Quality of movement**: Smooth, choppy, slippery, hesitant. This is where classical descriptions can sound strange until you feel them. A "slippery" pulse is not a metaphor—it's a tactile sense of continuous, rounded movement. "Choppy" is not judgment; it's the feeling of unevenness, like a wheel with missing spokes.
- **Coherence**: Does the pulse feel integrated, as if the system is speaking with one voice? Or does it feel like competing signals—strong in one place, weak in another; floating and empty; fast but forceless? Coherence is one of the most clinically useful things to feel, and one of the hardest to quantify.

These qualities matter because they help you answer a question that is easy to miss in symptom-based thinking:

What is the body trying to do?

Is it trying to push something out? Hold something in? Compensate for depletion with tension? Keep circulation moving despite dryness? Stay functional despite cold? The pulse is often the fastest way to sense the strategy beneath the complaint.

A Clinical Moment: When the Pulse Changes the Story

A patient comes in for headaches. They describe them as tension headaches—band-like, worse with stress, better with heat. They've tried magnesium, physical therapy, and better posture. Helpful, but incomplete.

You might expect a tense, wiry pulse—something that echoes muscle tone and stress.

But imagine instead you find a pulse that is **thin**, **slightly rapid**, and **weak at depth**—especially in positions that correspond to fluids and restorative capacity. The tongue is slightly red, with little coat. The patient wakes thirsty, and their sleep is light. The headaches worsen late afternoon.

Now the story shifts. It's not only "tension." It's tension in a body that is slightly under-lubricated, under-rested, and running warm. Muscle tone becomes a compensation, not the root.

Treatment changes, too. You may still address tension. But you stop treating the case as a purely mechanical issue and start treating it as a regulatory problem: restore fluids, calm heat, support sleep depth and reduce the body's need to brace itself.

A month later, the patient says, "The headaches are less frequent, but also my sleep is deeper—and I didn't realize that was related."

That's the pulse doing what it does best: linking symptoms to strategy.

The Tongue as a Record of Transformation

If the pulse is conversation, the tongue is a ledger.

It's tempting to treat tongue diagnosis like a snapshot—take a look, match it to a chart, decide what it means. That's how it's often taught in simplified form. But the tongue is more valuable as a **record over time**.

Because the tongue changes slowly compared to moment-to-moment sensations, and because it reflects the state of fluids, digestion, heat dynamics, and tissue quality in a way that is visible.

In practice, the tongue is less like a "diagnosis" and more like a timeline:

- What has been brewing for months?
- What has been depleted gradually?
- What is stuck, and for how long?
- What has the body failed to fully transform and transport?
- What kind of heat has been quietly accumulating?

You can sometimes see the history of an illness on the tongue even when symptoms are currently muted—either because the patient has adapted, or because exogenous interventions are masking the subjective symptoms.

What We Look At–And Why It Matters

Again, specificity matters. Tongue diagnosis gets dismissed when it's spoken about vaguely. So here's what a clinician is actually looking at:

- **Body color**: pale, red, purple, or normal. Color can reflect temperature dynamics, blood movement, and the presence of heat or stagnation.
- **Shape and substance**: swollen, thin, scalloped edges, cracked, stiff. Shape tells you about fluids, tissue tone,

and chronicity. Scalloping can suggest swelling and poor transformation; thinness can suggest depletion. Cracks can indicate long-term dryness or heat patterns—not always pathological, but meaningful in context.

- **Coating**: thickness, color, texture, distribution, and whether it's rooted. Coating can reflect the state of digestion, fluids, and what classical texts call "turbidity" or "dampness." A greasy coat is different from a dry coat; a thick coat that is peeled in patches (a geographic tongue) is different from a uniform thin coat. These distinctions matter because they indicate different physiological bottlenecks.
- **Moisture**: wet, normal, dry. Moisture tells you quickly whether fluids are adequate and whether heat is consuming them.
- **Movement**: Does the tongue extend easily? Is it rigid? Does it tremble? Is the person able to show it without strain? These are subtle but can correlate with neurological tone, anxiety, internal wind patterns, or depletion.

But here's the key: none of these features "mean" anything in isolation. A pale tongue could be cold, could be a deficiency, could be constitutional. A red tongue could be heat, could be emotion, could be diet, could be medication. The meaning emerges when the tongue is read alongside pulse, symptoms, history, and the person's baseline.

The tongue is not a verdict. It's a clue that has weight because it is relatively hard to fake.

A Tongue That Tells the Truth When the Patient Can't Yet

Sometimes patients are articulate and precise. Sometimes they're exhausted, overwhelmed, or have lived in their symptoms for so long that they can't tell you what's normal anymore.

They'll say, "I'm fine." Or: "It's just stress."

And you look at the tongue and see a red tip, dry coat, maybe cracks, maybe a peeled area. Or you see a thick, greasy coat and swollen body, and the patient says they "eat pretty clean." Or you see a purple hue and distended sublingual veins, and the patient is describing pain that "moves around."

This isn't about catching anyone in a lie. It's about the limits of self-report.

Humans normalize their suffering. They adapt. They forget what rested feels like. They confuse "functional" with "well." The tongue sometimes reveals what the person has been living with quietly.

And then the work is not to announce what you see like a fortune teller. The work is to translate it into useful next steps:

- "Your body looks like it's running a bit warm and dry. That would fit with the light sleep and afternoon crashes."
- "There are signs your digestion is working harder than it should. Let's talk about stool, appetite, and what happens after meals."
- "Your circulation looks constrained. Let's track pain patterns and temperature changes."

The tongue helps you ask better questions.

Transformation Over Time: Why Follow-Up Matters

One of the most underappreciated aspects of tongue diagnosis is that it can show you whether your treatment is changing the terrain, even before symptoms fully resolve.

A thick coat gradually thinning—not disappearing overnight, but shifting steadily—can suggest that digestion and fluid metabolism are improving. A tongue that is dry and red, then gains a thin, moist coat, can suggest that fluids are being restored and heat is dissipating. A purple tongue that becomes more pink can suggest improved circulation and reduced stagnation.

These changes are not always linear. Sometimes the tongue looks "worse" for a week as the body mobilizes and clears. Sometimes symptoms improve before the tongue changes, because the nervous system calms faster than the deeper physiology rebuilds. Sometimes the tongue improves while symptoms lag behind, especially in long-standing chronic cases where the body needs time to trust the new conditions.

That's why the tongue is a record. It keeps you honest. It prevents you from treating only the current flare. It reminds you that healing is often a sequence of reorganizations, not a straight line.

Why These Methods Require Training, Not Belief

If you've ever watched someone learn wine tasting or music theory, you've seen this phenomenon: at first, everything tastes like "wine," and everything sounds like "music." Over time, the senses differentiate. You learn to perceive what was always there.

Pulse and tongue are like that. They require **calibration**.

Belief is not the point. In fact, belief can get in the way because it makes people reach for certainty too quickly. The real skill is to hold your perception lightly but clearly: to feel what you feel, to see what you see, and to check it against outcomes.

Training matters for several reasons:

1. **Your hands lie at first.** Not because they're dishonest, but because they're untrained. A beginner presses too hard, or too lightly, or can't maintain a consistent depth. They confuse their own nervousness with the patient's pulse.
2. **Language can mislead.** Words like "slippery" and "wiry" are useful within a shared tactile culture, but they're not self-explanatory. Without supervised practice, students attach the wrong sensations to the words and build a shaky diagnostic vocabulary.

3. **Pattern recognition is earned, not imagined.** The pulse quality that indicates constraint in one body may indicate pain in another, and anxiety in a third. The mapping is not one-to-one. It's one-to-many, filtered through context. That's why apprenticeship matters.
4. **Confirmation bias is real.** If you want to feel a "Kidney deficiency pulse" badly enough, you will. If you expect every stressed person to have a wiry pulse, you'll find wiry everywhere. Training has to include learning how you fool yourself.

Good training doesn't make you omniscient. It makes you **reliable**.

And reliability in this context means: your observations lead to decisions that help, and your confidence stays proportional to the evidence.

Why Instruments Can't Replace Cultivated Perception

It might sound like we're setting up a rivalry: ancient hands versus modern machines. That's not the point. We've already acknowledged the miracle of modern anatomy and imaging. When you need surgery, you need surgery. When you need a scan, you need a scan.

The real question is narrower and more practical:

Why can't we just measure whatever the pulse and tongue are supposedly telling us?

We can measure some of it. Heart rate variability, blood pressure, oxygen saturation, inflammatory markers, thyroid hormones, microbiome data, sleep stages, glucose curves, and skin temperature. These are valuable.

But the pulse and tongue aren't primarily about data quantity. They're about **integration**.

A machine can give you one channel with high precision. A trained clinician can perceive multiple channels at once—not with the same precision, but with an ability to sense coherence, compensation, and directionality.

Let me say that more plainly:

- Instruments are excellent at *isolating variables.*
- Cultivated perception is good at *reading the whole organism in context.*

And that context includes things machines don't easily capture:

- how symptoms cluster
- how the body responds to touch and attention
- the timing of changes across a day
- the relationship between stress and digestion, or sleep and pain
- the difference between high energy and high tension
- the difference between "inflammation" as a lab value and "heat" as a lived physiology

There's also the fact that instruments don't interpret themselves. Data still requires a mind. And minds still rely on pattern recognition. The question becomes: what patterns are you trained to see?

A clinician with cultivated perception is not anti-measurement. They're anti-replacement.

Because if you replace perception with numbers alone, you risk losing the ability to detect what patients feel most: shifts in resilience, adaptability, and internal stability—changes that often precede or outlast the lab abnormalities.

The Limits of Pulse and Tongue—and How Good Physicians Compensate

If pulse and tongue were perfect, we wouldn't need the rest of the clinical encounter. We could diagnose behind a curtain. Some traditions flirted with that fantasy. It doesn't hold up in real life.

Pulse and tongue have limits. Naming those limits is part of practicing honesty.

Limit 1: They Are Not Specific to Disease Names

Pulse and tongue don't tell you "endometriosis" or "Hashimoto's" or "ulcerative colitis." They tell you about terrain: heat, cold, constraint, deficiency, fluid status, circulation quality, and the body's current regulatory strategy.

That can be profoundly useful, but it does not replace biomedical diagnosis where biomedical diagnosis matters—especially when red flags are present.

Compensation: A responsible clinician screens for red flags, refers when needed, and collaborates with biomedical assessment rather than competing with it. Pulse and tongue help guide supportive care and pattern-based treatment; they do not excuse you from basic safety.

Limit 2: They Are Influenced by Temporary Conditions

The pulse changes with caffeine, a stressful commute, a night of poor sleep, dehydration, exercise, medications, a recent meal, and even the emotional intensity of visiting a clinician.

The tongue changes with coffee, food dyes, brushing, smoking, and acute illness. It also changes more slowly than symptoms in some cases, and more quickly in others.

Compensation: You ask about context before you interpret. You recheck. You track over time. You don't make grand claims from one reading. You treat pulse and tongue as living signals, not fixed labels.

Limit 3: The Clinician Is Part of the Instrument

Your fingers have temperature. Your attention has steadiness or distraction. Your own nervous system entrains with the patient. This is not mystical; it's physiology and psychology. Two bodies in proximity influence each other.

A clinician who is rushed will miss things. A clinician who is anxious will apply techniques sloppily. A clinician trying to impress will overinterpret.

Compensation: You train. You slow down. You standardize your method. You check yourself. Good clinicians develop rituals of attention—not for drama, but to reduce noise in the measurement.

Limit 4: They Can Be Ambiguous

Some pulses are clear. Some are muddy. Some tongues are textbook. Some are confusing. And sometimes the signals disagree: the pulse says heat, the tongue says cold; the symptoms say deficiency, the pulse says excess.

This is where simplistic teaching fails, because students expect consistency. Real bodies are not obligated to be consistent.

Ambiguity often means one of three things:

1. The body is in transition.
2. The case is layered (for example: deficiency underneath, constraint on top).
3. You're missing key context.

Compensation: You widen the data set. You palpate the abdomen. You check temperature, skin quality, and muscle tone. You listen for timing patterns. You ask about thirst, urination, bowel movements, sleep architecture, and emotional triggers. You may do a short course of treatment as a diagnostic probe: if you move the constraint and the pulse softens, that tells you something. If you tonify and the person feels worse, that tells you something, too.

Good clinicians don't pretend ambiguity isn't there. They work with it.

What Physicians Perceive That Patients Rarely Notice

There's a moment in many appointments where a patient looks at me, watching their tongue or feeling their pulse and asks—sometimes aloud, sometimes silently—*What could you possibly know from that?*

Here's one answer: I'm often tracking **direction** more than I'm tracking diagnosis.

In chronic illness, the most important question is not "What do you have?" but:

Is your body becoming more capable of regulating itself?

That's not a philosophical question. It shows up in very concrete ways:

- Does your sleep become deeper, even if it isn't perfect?
- Does your digestion become less reactive?
- Does your pain become less sticky and less unpredictable?
- Do you recover faster after stress?
- Does your mood become less brittle?
- Does your cycle become more regular, less clotty, less symptomatic?

- Do you feel warmer in a healthy way, rather than inflamed?

- Does your pulse become more rooted, more even, more coherent?

- Does your tongue regain moisture and a stable coat?

These are not glamorous outcomes. They don't always fit into a before-and-after post. But they are often the real signs that a system is reorganizing toward health.

Pulse and tongue help you perceive those subtle shifts early—sometimes before the patient trusts them, sometimes before the lab values budge, sometimes before the symptoms fully relent.

The Quiet Difference Between Certainty and Clarity

People crave certainty in medicine for good reasons. When you're suffering, uncertainty feels like danger. When you're responsible for someone's care, uncertainty can feel irresponsible, like you're letting the patient down.

But certainty is not always available. And chasing it can make clinicians dishonest—either by overpromising, or by clinging to a single explanation when the case is complex.

Classical methods—pulse and tongue included—live in a different posture. They don't promise certainty. They aim for clarity.

Clarity looks like this:

- We may not know the final diagnosis today, but we can see that your system is running hot and dry, and we can start changing that.

- We may not be able to prove, in one visit, why your digestion and anxiety are linked, but the pulse shows tension, the tongue shows stagnation, the history shows timing patterns, and treating that network is reasonable.

- We may not be able to guarantee the outcome, but we can track whether the body is moving toward coherence or away from it.

Clarity is not vague. It's specific about what is known, what is suspected, what is dangerous, and what is actionable.

And it's humble about what remains uncertain.

That posture—honest, observant, iterative—is where this medicine becomes most powerful. Not as an alternative mythology, but as a disciplined way of listening to the living body.

Closing: Learning to Hear What the Body Is Already Saying

Pulse and tongue diagnosis are often portrayed as mysterious because the culture around them sometimes becomes theatrical. But in their best form, they are not theater. They are **craft**.

They ask something of the clinician: patience, sensory refinement, willingness to be wrong, and willingness to learn from follow-up. And they offer something to the patient: a form of attention that doesn't reduce their experience to a single organ or a single lab value.

In a world where medical encounters are increasingly compressed, there is something quietly radical about taking the body seriously as a communicating system.

Not because it makes us certain.

Because even without certainty, we can still have clarity—and clarity is enough to begin.

6

Constitution and Temporality

One of the first disappointments for anyone who wants medicine to be clean and predictable is this: two people can have the same diagnosis, the same lab values, the same lifestyle on paper, and still respond in completely different ways.

One person gets sick, rests for a weekend, and returns to baseline as if nothing happened. Another gets sick and never quite returns—months later, they're still "not right." A third doesn't crash dramatically at all. They just slowly narrow: less resilience, less range, less enthusiasm. They don't fall apart; they stagnate.

If you've lived inside a chronic condition—or treated enough of them—you stop asking, "What is *the* disease?" and start asking, "What is *this person's* relationship to stress, time, and repair?"

Classical Chinese medicine has a word for that relationship: **constitution**. But the constitution isn't fate or a personality test. It's a clinical way of describing how a particular body tends to distribute its resources, where it compensates first, and what it pays for that compensation over the years.

And then there's the other half of the equation—often missed even by experienced clinicians: **temporality**. Not just "how long has this been going on?" but *what phase is this person in*, and what does this phase allow?

The same pattern at twenty-five and at sixty is not the same pattern. The same insomnia in the first month after childbirth and five years into perimenopause is not the same insomnia. The same "fatigue" after a divorce and after a decade of caregiving is not the same fatigue. The body is the body—but it is never the same body twice.

This chapter is about how we think in light of those realities.

A PERSON IS NOT A DIAGNOSIS; THEY ARE A CONFIGURATION

In clinic, I'm often meeting people at a moment of betrayal. Their body isn't doing what it used to do, and they want to know why. They've read the lists. They've tried the supplements. They've wondered if it's their hormones, their thyroid, their gut, their trauma, their nervous system, or their mindset.

Usually, it's not one thing.

What I'm looking for is a *configuration*: a particular arrangement of strengths and vulnerabilities that has been there for a long time—sometimes since childhood—combined with whatever has happened recently that tipped the system into a new mode.

Constitution, in this sense, is not a single trait ("yin deficient," "liver qi stagnation"). It's more like a **bias** in the organism:

- Where do they generate power easily, and where do they struggle?
- Do they run hot under pressure or go cold?
- When stressed, do they tighten and push harder, or collapse and withdraw?
- Do they tend toward dryness or dampness, tension or looseness, volatility or flatness?
- Do symptoms move quickly, or do they settle in and become fixed?

In Chinese medicine language, we're watching the interplay of **qi, blood, fluids, yin, yang**, and the deeper reserve we call **jing**. But the point isn't to label someone like a specimen. The point is to predict how their system behaves over time and what kinds of interventions it can actually use.

You can give the same herb to two people and watch opposite outcomes—not because herbs are magical, but because physiology is conditional. One person takes a warming formula and finally feels awake and functional; another becomes irritable, inflamed, and sleepless. The formula didn't "work" or "not work." The organism expressed it through its own configuration.

So constitution is not a diagnosis. It's the *terrain* in which the diagnosis is happening.

CONSTITUTIONAL TENDENCIES VERSUS SITUATIONAL IMBALANCE

Here's a question that comes up quietly in every intake, whether the patient asks it directly or not:

"Is this who I am, or is this something that happened to me?"

It matters because it shapes hope. If a symptom feels constitutional—"I've always been like this"—people tend to either resign themselves or overidentify with it. If it feels situational—"This started after X"—they want it gone, cleanly, like removing a splinter.

Clinically, the answer is usually: **both**.

There are **constitutional tendencies**, and there are **situational imbalances** that can overlay, distort, or exploit them.

A simple example: two people catch a virus.

- One person gets a fever, sweats, sleeps, and recovers. Their system knows how to *resolve* an acute event.
- Another person doesn't mount much fever, stays cold, appetite disappears, and weeks later, they're still

exhausted. Their system doesn't mobilize well, and the aftermath lingers.

The virus is the situational factor. The difference is constitutional. Not in a mystical sense—more like baseline immune responsiveness, autonomic tone, endocrine reserve, digestive capacity, sleep architecture, and recovery bandwidth.

Or take stress.

One person under stress becomes restless, wired, and angry. Another becomes foggy, heavy, and depressed. Another becomes compulsively productive and then crashes. These aren't moral differences. They're different default strategies of a system trying to maintain coherence.

A situational imbalance is often more *reversible*. It has a clearer onset, a sharper edge. It may respond quickly when the right lever is pulled—sleep restored, inflammation reduced, digestion stabilized, acute grief metabolized.

A constitutional tendency tends to be more *persistent*. It may soften and mature, but it rarely disappears entirely. A person with a lifelong tendency toward dryness may always have to respect hydration and rest more than their friends. A person with a naturally "hot" system may always need to be careful with stimulants, alcohol, and overtraining. A person with weak digestive transformation may always need to eat more simply than the foodie culture would like.

The mistake is to treat constitutional tendencies as unchangeable *and* to treat situational imbalances as trivial.

The more accurate view is:

- **The current Constitution sets the strengths and weaknesses of the system.**
- **The Situation determines how hard the system is being asked to work, and in what way.**
- **Time shows the adaptive potential of the combination of the two.**

WHY SOME PEOPLE BREAK UNDER STRESS WHILE OTHERS STAGNATE

People tend to imagine stress as a universal toxin. More stress equals more symptoms. Reducing stress equals recovery. If only.

Stress is not just a load. Stress is also *how the system is organized to meet the load.*

When two people face the same pressure—work deadlines, caregiving, financial strain—one may "break" dramatically: panic attacks, insomnia, palpitations, autoimmune flares, migraines, dysautonomia. Another may not break. They may simply lose motion: weight creeps up, libido fades, digestion dulls, mood flattens, joints stiffen, cycles become irregular. They don't fall off a cliff. They slowly stop climbing.

In Chinese medicine terms, both are forms of dysregulation, but they're shaped differently by constitutional bias and by the phase of life.

The "break" pattern: brittle compensation

Some people hold themselves together with high-tension strategies. Their system compensates through mobilization—sympathetic drive, adrenaline, cortisol rhythms that look "fine" until they don't. They often appear functional right up to the moment they aren't.

These are the patients who say things like:

- "I can handle a lot, until suddenly I can't."
- "I used to run on stress."
- "I don't feel tired until bedtime, then I can't sleep."

Their body isn't weak in the obvious way. It's strong in a narrow channel, and fragile outside it. The compensation is effective but expensive.

In classical language, you might see **liver qi constraint transforming into heat**, **heart agitation**, **yin damage from prolonged hyperarousal**, or **qi and blood not returning**

inward. But the lived reality is simpler: the system has been running too close to its redline, and it loses its ability to downshift.

When these patients crash, they often interpret it as failure. But clinically, the crash can be a kind of forced reorganization—painful, disruptive, but sometimes necessary. The danger is not the crash itself. The danger is trying to climb back into the same brittle structure that produced it.

The "stagnation" pattern: heavy compensation

Other people meet stress by conserving. Their system slows output, stores more, moves less, digests more poorly, and thinks more slowly. They may not panic; they may simply become less alive.

They often say:

- "I don't feel anxious. I just don't care."
- "I wake up tired and stay tired."
- "My body feels heavy."
- "Nothing is terribly wrong, but nothing is right either."

In Chinese medicine, we often see **spleen qi weakness**, **damp accumulation**, **phlegm misting**, or **yang not moving fluids**. Again, the labels matter less than the recognition: the body has chosen a low-power mode. It may be protecting itself from depletion, inflammation and repeated overstimulation. But that protection has a cost—circulation, clarity, desire, and flexibility decline.

These are the patients who can go years without a dramatic event, and then look back and realize their health has decreased, that they've aged dramatically in a short time.

Same stress, different math

So why do these two patterns diverge?

Because stress is not just an external force. It's a negotiation between **demand** and **reserve**.

Two people can have the same demand. One has more reserve, or more efficient recovery, or fewer leaks in the system. Another has hidden deficits—sleep debt, metabolic fragility, unresolved inflammation, poor digestion, long-term grief. The same stressor lands differently because it lands on different terrain.

This is where constitution meets temporality: a strategy that worked at twenty-five may fail at forty-five—not because the patient aged, but because, as they aged, they did so in a way which made them brittle.

AGE, HISTORY, AND INHERITANCE: THE LONG ARC INSIDE THE SYMPTOM

Chinese medicine has always been comfortable talking about inheritance without pretending to know everything about it. The classical idea of **pre-heaven essence (jing)** is a way of acknowledging that we are born with a certain allotment: not a fixed lifespan, but a baseline of health: repair capacity, endocrine reserve, developmental robustness, and resilience.

Modern language gives us genetics, epigenetics, prenatal environment, childhood adversity, microbiome inheritance, and more. Different vocabulary, similar humility: you don't get to choose your starting point.

But inheritance is only the first layer. The second is history—the accumulated record of what your body has had to do to survive your life.

The body remembers in practical ways.

When I say "history," I don't mean a story you tell in therapy—though that can matter too. I mean the body's practical adaptations:

- Years of night shift work reshaping circadian hormones
- Repeated dieting changing metabolic efficiency
- Chronic inflammation altering vascular tone and sleep depth

- Long-term anxiety training the respiratory diaphragm into a guarded pattern
- Repeated infections changing immune reactivity
- Pregnancy, breastfeeding, and postpartum depletion changing blood and fluid dynamics
- Concussions, surgeries, and anesthesia leaving subtle autonomic effects

These are not "trauma" as a buzzword. They're physiological facts.

A person's constitution is not just what they were born with. It's what they've become through adaptation.

Age isn't a number; it's a phase of resource strategy

Classical texts talk about life in cycles—often in seven-year increments for women and eight-year increments for men—not as rigid fate, but as a recognition that endocrine and reproductive rhythms shape the whole system.

In practice, what changes with age is not simply "decline." It's a shift in the body's budgeting.

In youth, the system is biased toward growth and outward motion. In midlife, it's biased toward maintenance and reproduction (whether or not one has children). Later, it's biased toward conservation and internal stabilization.

So symptoms that were once "minor" become meaningful. A little sleep loss in your twenties is annoying. The same sleep loss in your forties might trigger palpitations, reflux, mood volatility, or a flare of pain. Not because you're weaker in character, but because the margin is smaller and the consequences ripple wider.

Family patterns are clues, not verdicts

When someone tells me "everyone in my family has anxiety" or "autoimmune disease runs in our family," I don't hear doom. I hear a map.

Family patterns often point to constitutional tendencies: inflammatory bias, metabolic fragility, connective tissue laxity, migraine tendencies, mood reactivity, skin sensitivity, and digestive weakness.

The clinical question becomes: *Given this map, what is most preventable? What is most modifiable? What must be respected early rather than argued with later?*

Some of the best medicine is anticipatory. You don't wait for the crash to start building recovery capacity.

TEMPORALITY: PATTERNS ARE NOT STATIC; THEY EVOLVE

Earlier, we talked about chronic illness as something with phases, not a single story. Here's where that becomes practical.

A pattern that looks like "liver qi stagnation" in year one may look like "blood stasis" in year five—not because the diagnosis changed arbitrarily, but because *time crystallizes function into structure*. The body repeats what it has to repeat, and repetition leaves residue.

In clinic, you can often feel this difference:

- Early-stage problems are more *mobile*: symptoms fluctuate, respond to stress, and change with sleep.
- Later-stage problems are more *fixed*: pain localizes, cycles become entrenched, digestion loses flexibility, and mood becomes less responsive to context.

That doesn't mean early-stage problems are "easy." It means they're more plastic. The system is still negotiating. Later-stage problems may be stable but stubborn.

Temporality asks us to treat the person we have now, not the person they were at onset.

It also keeps us honest about expectations. Some things improve quickly; others improve slowly; others may not fully reverse but can be made livable, stable, and less costly.

WHY TREATMENT STRATEGIES SHIFT OVER TIME

Patients sometimes experience this as inconsistency:

"Last year, you said we should clear heat. Now you're tonifying."
"First, it was all about regulation. Now it's about strengthening."
"Why are we changing the plan if the diagnosis is the same?"

Because the plan is not a moral commitment. It's a response to a moving system.

There are a few common reasons for strategy changes.

1) The body's priorities change once survival is less urgent

In an acute flare—panic, insomnia, a pain spike, a colitis flare—the body is in emergency mode. If we treat only the long-term root and ignore the flare, we can lose the patient (or their trust). Sometimes you have to put out the fire so that the house can be repaired.

Once the flare is controlled, the deeper pattern becomes visible: the depletion, the poor recovery, the brittle stress response, the digestive weakness that made the fire easier to ignite.

So treatment shifts from **containment** to **rebuilding**.

2) You can't strengthen what is blocked, and you can't disperse forever

There's a simple clinical rhythm:

- If a system is constrained, congested, overheated, or inflamed, tonics can aggravate it.
- If a system is depleted, chronically dispersing can exhaust it further.

Early on, we may need to regulate—move, vent, harmonize. Later, we may need to consolidate—nourish, anchor, strengthen.

This isn't formula worship. It's resource logic.

3) The person changes as they learn about their own body

Treatment doesn't happen to a passive object. People adapt. They learn what makes them worse and what makes them better. They change food, sleep, boundaries, training, and work rhythms. That changes the physiology we're treating.

A good plan should evolve with the patient's capacity and insight.

4) Age and life stage change what "successful treatment" means

A twenty-eight-year-old with irregular cycles may want fertility support now. A forty-eight-year-old may want a less turbulent peri-menopause. A sixty-year-old may want pain-free walking and clear sleep. These are not the same goals, and they shouldn't be forced into the same strategy.

The medicine should meet the patient where they're at in their life.

CURING VERSUS CORRECTING: WHAT ARE WE ACTUALLY TRYING TO DO?

This is one of the most important conversations in the clinic, and it's often implied rather than spoken.

People come in wanting a cure. Of course they do. They want the thing gone. They want their old body back. They want certainty.

Sometimes, cure is realistic—especially when the problem is mostly situational, recent, and functionally driven. Sometimes what we can do is better described as **correction**: restoring function, reducing symptom intensity, widening tolerance, preventing progression, and building resilience.

Correction is not failure. It's a mature goal.

Here are a few ways I think about the difference.

Cure is the removal of a driver

If there is a clear driver—an exposure, an infection, a medication effect, a nutrient deficiency, a mechanical issue—then a cure can be possible if that driver is removed and the system can reset.

In Chinese medicine, this often corresponds to expelling a pathogen, clearing acute heat, resolving lodged dampness—*when the body still has the power to finish the job.*

Correction is re-patterning and support

When the condition is embedded in long-term physiology—years of poor sleep architecture, endocrine depletion, autonomic rigidity, longstanding digestive weakness, a constitutional bias towards inflammation—then the realistic target is often correction:

- fewer flares
- faster recovery
- better sleep depth
- improved digestion and energy stability
- less reactivity to stress
- more predictable cycles
- reduced reliance on brittle compensations (caffeine, adrenaline, overtraining, pain killers, etc.)

Correction is the art of making a life resilient again.

Sometimes "cure" is the wrong question

There are cases where the body has changed structurally—degenerative joint changes, certain neuropathies, tissue damage, or surgical removal of tissue. Then the goal becomes: **How do we reduce suffering and maximize function without lying to anyone?**

Chinese medicine can be powerful here, but not because it does something magical. It helps the remaining physiology do its job with less friction.

HOW CLINICIANS DECIDE WHAT CAN BE CHANGED AND WHAT MUST BE SUPPORTED

This is where clinical reasoning becomes intimate. Not sentimental—intimate in the sense that you're dealing with the person's actual constraints.

A clinician is always making a quiet triage:

- What is malleable right now?
- What is not malleable but can be buffered?
- What looks constitutional but is actually just long-standing compensation?
- What looks situational but is actually revealing a deeper fragility?

There isn't a single test for this. It's a way of thinking, built from observation over time.

1) Onset and trajectory: Did this arrive suddenly or gradually?

Sudden onset after a clear event (infection, grief, childbirth, move, injury) suggests a situational driver that may be reversible—at least partially.

Gradual onset over years suggests constitutional tendencies, long-term depletion, or cumulative dysregulation. Those can still improve, but they rarely flip quickly.

2) Variability: Does it fluctuate with context?

If symptoms change dramatically with sleep, stress, meals, weather, menstrual phase, or rest days, that's often a sign of functional dysregulation—more plastic, more responsive to intervention.

If symptoms are flat and unchanging regardless of context, that can suggest deeper structural change or entrenched regulation patterns. It can also mean the person has lost signal clarity—common in chronic fatigue states where the system's feedback loops are blunted.

3) Recovery signature: how does the person bounce back?

I ask questions like:

- If you overdo it, do you recover overnight, in three days, or in three weeks?
- After travel, how long until your digestion and sleep normalize?
- If you catch a cold, do you recover quickly, or does it linger and recur repeatedly without resolution?

These aren't casual questions. They're windows into reserve.

4) The cost of compensation: what is the body paying to function?

Earlier, we talked about compensations—the clever ways the body keeps you going. Clinically, I'm tracking what those compensations cost:

- High output sustained by stimulants → insomnia, palpitations, anxiety
- Tight musculoskeletal bracing → headaches, jaw tension, pelvic pain

- Digestive issues through poor diet → bloating, reflux, skin flares
- Emotional suppression → depression, fatigue, immune fragility
- Overtraining to manage mood → injuries, menstrual disruption, burnout

When we treat, we're not only trying to remove symptoms. We're trying to lower the cost of being functional.

5) What happens when we nudge the system?

Sometimes the most revealing thing is a gentle intervention.

A small dose of acupuncture, a modest formula, a simple sleep protocol—does the body soften? Does it stabilize? Or does it resist and rebound?

A system that can accept a nudge has room to change. A system that rebounds violently may need slower approaches, narrower aims, and more support before deeper shifts are possible.

This is also where clinician humility matters. If you push a fragile system too aggressively—whether by "detoxing," over-dispersing, over-tonifying, or insisting on lifestyle changes beyond capacity—you can create chaos. In theory, your fatigued patient may need stimulants. In practice, this approach may further disorder their system. The system must be able to integrate the intervention such that the patient moves towards resilience.

THE DEEPER CONSTITUTIONAL QUESTION: WHAT IS BEING PROTECTED?

Here's a subtle shift that often changes everything:

Instead of asking "What's wrong?" we ask, **"What is the body protecting, and at what cost?"**

A person who is always tense may be protecting against collapse. A person who is always tired may be protecting against overstimulation. A person with chronic dampness may be protecting against dryness and overheating. A person with insomnia may be protecting against feelings that surface when things get quiet.

This is not psychologizing physiology. It's recognizing that organisms choose strategies.

Classical Chinese medicine is unusually good at this because it never pretended the body was a machine with isolated parts. It assumes the body is a negotiating intelligence—sometimes wise, sometimes stuck, always trying to maintain coherence.

When we see symptoms as protective strategies, we stop fighting them blindly. We start asking what would make the protection unnecessary.

TIME AS A CLINICAL TOOL: PACING, SEQUENCE, AND PATIENCE

Temporality isn't just descriptive. It becomes a tool.

Sequence matters

If someone is deeply depleted but also inflamed and congested, you can't simply "tonify the deficiency." You may need to first open pathways, reduce friction, restore sleep, and improve digestion so nourishment can actually be used.

If someone is brittle and anxious with insomnia, you may need to first anchor and settle before you try to "move stagnation," or you'll stir the system into more agitation.

In other words: you don't treat the textbook. You treat the order in which the body can safely change.

Pacing is medicine

People often underestimate pacing because it sounds like lifestyle advice. But pacing is a direct intervention in autonomic and immune regulation.

If a person with post-viral fatigue keeps trying to "push through," no formula will overcome that mismatch. Conversely, if someone with stagnation never moves their body or takes emotional risks, acupuncture may create movement but won't create momentum.

Pacing is the bridge between constitution and time: it respects reserve while slowly expanding it.

Patience isn't passive

There's a kind of patience that is resignation, and a kind that is strategy.

When we aim for correction rather than cure, patience becomes active: we make small changes that compound. We watch which changes hold. We back off when the system protests. We advance when it opens.

Over months, this can create a stability that feels—subjectively—like getting one's life back.

WHAT IT LOOKS LIKE IN A REAL CLINIC

Let me give you a few composite portraits—real patterns, with identifying details removed.

The high-functioning collapse

A woman in her late thirties comes in after a year of insomnia and palpitations. She used to be "the energetic one." She exercises hard, runs a team at work, drinks coffee, eats "clean," and prides herself on mental toughness. The symptoms started after a promotion and a family illness—more responsibility, less rest.

Constitutionally, she runs warm, tends toward tension, and has always been a light sleeper. Situationally, she has been in a prolonged state of mobilization.

If I treat only the "stress" (tell her to relax), she feels blamed. If I treat only the symptoms (sedate, suppress), she feels temporarily better but loses function.

The strategy shifts over time:

1. **Stabilize sleep and palpitations** (anchor, settle, reduce internal agitation).
2. **Restore recovery capacity** (build yin/blood, improve digestion so nourishment lands).
3. **Unwind the long-held tension pattern** (gentle movement of constraint, not aggressive dispersal).
4. **Teach pacing that doesn't feel like failure** (so she can stop paying for productivity with her nervous system).

This is not a quick cure. But correction can be profound: she becomes someone who can be strong without being brittle. She can build her relationship with her system so that she knows when she's becoming dysregulated and can make conscious choices about how to respond.

The slow narrowing

A man in his fifties comes in with weight gain, brain fog, low libido, and joint stiffness. He isn't anxious. He's "fine." But he feels older than his age. The onset was gradual over a decade of desk work, poor sleep, alcohol with dinner, and chronic worry, which he doesn't name as worry.

Constitutionally, he tends toward dampness and sluggish digestion. Situationally, his life has been low-movement, high-responsibility, low-joy.

If I push too hard—strong cleansing, aggressive exercise demands—he rebounds, gets sore, quits, and concludes nothing works.

The time-aware strategy is different:

1. **Lighten without draining** (support digestion, reduce damp accumulation gently).
2. **Reintroduce circulation** in a way that his joints and sleep can tolerate.

3. **Build yang function slowly** (not with stimulants, but with steady rhythm, morning light, consistent meals, appropriate warming support).
4. **Measure success by range**: he doesn't need to become twenty-five. He needs to become more himself again.

The inherited edge

A young adult with a family history of autoimmune conditions develops eczema, digestive sensitivity, and anxiety in college. The body is reactive; symptoms flare with exams and poor sleep.

Here, the constitutional inflammatory bias matters. But so does temporality: early intervention can prevent deeper embedding.

Treatment is partly symptom control, but the larger aim is teaching the body a different relationship to stress and recovery. This is where Chinese medicine can be quietly preventative—if it's used to build resilience rather than chase every flare like a whack-a-mole game.

THE ETHICS OF REALISM: HOPE WITHOUT FANTASY

Patients can feel crushed when a clinician implies something is constitutional—as if they're being told, "This is just you."

But there's another kind of harm: offering cure fantasies to someone whose body needs a longer, slower kind of repair.

A mature clinical relationship holds both:

- **Respect for what is real and constrained**
- **Curiosity about what is still changeable**

Often, the most meaningful improvements come not from forcing change where the system can't comply, but from finding the lever that allows change to occur naturally.

Sometimes that lever is sleep. Sometimes it's digestion. Sometimes it's grief. Sometimes it's reducing overtraining. Sometimes it's warmth and regular meals. Sometimes it's finally treating pain that has been driving sympathetic tone for years.

The art is not in having the fanciest tools. It's in choosing the right sequence, at the right pace, for this specific body at this specific time.

CLOSING: THE BODY YOU HAVE, THE TIME YOU'RE IN

Constitution is the hand you were dealt, plus the way you've learned to play it. Temporality is the game clock—the phase you're in, the momentum you carry, the debts that have accrued, the reserves you can draw on.

When we bring these together, medicine becomes less performative and more honest.

We stop asking only, "What do you have?" and start asking:

- What has your body been doing for you?
- What has it been paying to do it?
- What is still negotiable?
- What needs support before it can change?
- What does healing mean at this stage of your life?
- What would you do if you were free of this problem?

Those questions don't produce simplistic answers. But they produce something better: coherent decisions.

And in complex chronic illness, coherence is not a luxury. It's the beginning of repair.

7

Acupuncture as Regulation

The most common story about acupuncture goes something like this: a practitioner stimulates a point, the nervous system responds, and symptoms improve. It's not wrong. It's just incomplete in the way most true-but-small explanations are incomplete.

In a clinic, acupuncture rarely behaves like a simple on–off switch. If it did, we could standardize it the way we standardize a light fixture: same wiring, same switch, same outcome. Instead, acupuncture acts more like a conversation with a living system—one that answers back, sometimes clearly, sometimes indirectly, sometimes with a delay. The needle is not the message by itself. The message is the *relationship* between the needle, the tissue, the timing, the patient's current state, and the clinician's intent.

When acupuncture works well, it doesn't feel like we're "adding something" to the body. It feels like we're helping the body *find its own settings again*—temperature, pressure, tone, rhythm, digestion, sleep. Regulation. Not in a vague, mystical way, but in the practical way you notice when a person walks in wired and leaves quieter; when a migraine pattern loses its predictability; when a shoulder that has been guarding for months finally lets go without being forced.

This chapter is about that regulatory view: acupuncture as communication rather than stimulation, why precision matters more than quantity, and why the results depend as much on perception as on point selection. It's also about limits—because any honest medicine needs a chapter about when it *shouldn't* be used—and a detour into "dry needling," which is often presented as a modern invention but is, in many ways, an ancient technique wearing new clothes.

Acupuncture as Communication with the Body, Not Stimulation

The language we use shapes what we look for. If you think acupuncture is primarily stimulation, you'll tend to measure success in terms of intensity: stronger sensation, more needles, more "treatment." If you think acupuncture is communication, you'll measure success in terms of *response*: softer breath, warmer hands, a change in facial color, a pulse that normalizes, a spasm that releases, a mind that becomes less hypervigilant.

Communication implies two things that "stimulation" quietly ignores:

1. **The body has context.**
2. The same input does not mean the same thing on different days. Touch a bruise and the message is "danger." Touch a tense shoulder, and the message might be "support" or "threat" depending on how it's done and how safe the person feels.
3. **The body interprets.**
4. A needle isn't a command; it's information. The system decides what to do with it. Sometimes the most useful information is not "do more," but "stop overdoing." Sometimes it's not "move the stagnation," but "hold the boundary."

Classical texts often describe acupuncture in terms that can sound foreign—"moving Qi," "regulating the channels," "harmonizing"—but the clinical experience underneath those words is surprisingly concrete. You place a needle, and the body reorganizes around it. Sometimes it does it immediately. Sometimes it resists. Sometimes it overshoots, and you have to back off. The practitioner isn't an electrician wiring a circuit; they're closer to a pilot making tiny adjustments in changing weather. This is part of why negative responses are so rare; we're not overriding the body, we're in dialogue with it.

That's why a good treatment doesn't feel like a pincushion. It feels like an intelligent intervention: a few points that speak clearly, rather than many points that talk over each other.

Why Precision Matters More Than Quantity

There's a stage many practitioners go through—especially early on—where more feels safer. If you're not sure what's happening, you add points. If you're not sure what to choose, you cover categories: something local, something distal, something calming, something "for the immune system." You build a net and hope the fish swim into it.

Sometimes they do. But often the net catches everything *except* the thing you were trying to change.

Precision matters because acupuncture is not just about *what* you needle. It's about *what you are asking the system to do*. And the more you ask at once, the less clear the request becomes.

Think of a patient with chronic headaches. You can needle the head, neck, hands, feet and ears; add cupping and electrostimulation; send them home with supplements, and it might still not change the pattern. Or you can find one or two points that reliably shift the autonomic tone—where the shoulders drop, the jaw releases, the eyes stop straining—and suddenly the headache becomes less "inevitable."

In those cases, the difference wasn't "more stimulation." It was *a clearer signal*.

There's also a physiological reality: every needle is a micro-injury. It's a controlled, tiny one, but it's still something the body has to process. A robust patient with good reserves might tolerate twenty needles and leave feeling great. A patient who is depleted, sensitive, or inflamed might leave foggy, shaky, or irritable from the same number. The question isn't "How many needles can I get away with?" It's "What is the smallest intervention that creates the right shift?"

A useful rule of thumb in the clinic is that when you find the right points, you often need fewer of them. When you're not sure, you tend to use more. More needles can hide uncertainty. Precision exposes it.

And precision is not an aesthetic preference. It's respect for the patient's system.

Depth, Angle, and Timing as Expressions of Intent

People talk about "acupuncture points" as if they're buttons on a flat surface. But the body isn't flat, and a point isn't a dot. It's a three-dimensional access route through layers: skin, fascia, muscle and neurovascular planes. When you change depth and angle, you change which layer you're communicating with. And that changes the message.

A shallow insertion can be enough to change the tone of the superficial tissues, especially in someone whose system is already reactive. A deeper insertion might reach a muscle plane that's been holding a pattern for years. An oblique angle might glide along fascia; a perpendicular angle might engage a deeper motor point. These are not merely technical variations—they're different communication systems which require different dialects.

Timing matters too, and not in a vague "energetic" sense. Timing includes:

- **The patient's breathing.**
- A needle placed as a patient exhales often lands differently than one placed as they inhale. If you've ever tried to relax a tight diaphragm or a guarded abdomen,

you learn quickly that breath is not a background detail —it's the gatekeeper.

- **The moment in the treatment.**
- Sometimes the first needle should be one that helps the system feel safe: a point that downshifts vigilance, settles the chest, or softens the face. Other times, you need to open a stuck area first, because the calm won't "take" until the pressure has an outlet. The order becomes part of the prescription.
- **How long the needle stays.**
- Retention time is dosage. Some patterns respond to brief, precise contact. Others need time—especially those involving chronic guarding—because the tissue doesn't trust the change yet. Leaving needles in longer isn't automatically better; it's simply another variable you can use with intent.
- **Whether you manipulate the needle.**
- There are times when you want to elicit a clear, strong tissue response—what many traditions call "arrival of Qi," and what a patient might describe as heaviness, dull ache, spreading warmth, or a pulling sensation. There are other times when you want almost none of that, because the person is already in a state of alarm. In those cases, forcing sensation is like raising your voice at someone who's already overwhelmed.

The deeper point here is that technique is not separate from diagnosis. Depth, angle, timing, and manipulation are part of the clinician's language. Two practitioners can needle the "same points" and deliver entirely different treatments because they spoke in different ways.

This is also why acupuncture is hard to study using simplistic protocols. If you reduce acupuncture to point names and ignore how the points were accessed—how the body was addressed—you end up researching a shadow of the real thing.

The Difference Between Locating a Point and Accessing It

Most people assume that if you can find the correct anatomical spot, you've "done the point." In practice, finding the spot is the beginning.

Locating a point is geometry. Accessing it is physiology.

A point can be technically correct and clinically dead. You can needle right where the textbook says and get nothing—not because acupuncture "doesn't work," but because you didn't actually enter the conversation.

Access involves a few elements that don't show up on charts:

- **Tissue quality.**
- Some points feel open and responsive; others feel bound, thickened, or oddly empty. Those qualities change with stress, inflammation, trauma, and chronic compensation. A point is not just a coordinate; it's a condition.
- **Palpatory listening.**
- Before the needle even touches the skin, a skilled clinician is gathering information: temperature, moisture, tone, tenderness and subtle pulsations. This isn't mysticism. It's pattern recognition with the hands. You learn what "normal" feels like in a thousand bodies, and you start noticing when something is not normal.
- **The patient's state of guarding or trust.**
- A point in a relaxed body is not the same point in a braced body. In one, the needle enters like a suggestion. In the other, it enters like an intrusion. Sometimes the first job of the treatment is not to "treat the condition," but to reduce the guarding enough for treatment to be even possible.
- **Micro-adjustments.**
- A millimeter matters. This surprises people. But when you're working near a fascial plane or a neurovascular bundle, a millimeter changes the conversation. You can

> be "on the point" and still be slightly off the structure that needs to be engaged. The difference often shows up immediately: a sensation that spreads versus one that stays sharp and local; a muscle that releases versus one that tightens.

In classical practice, this distinction is sometimes described as the difference between "knowing the point" and "meeting the Qi." In modern terms, it's the difference between treating a map and treating a person.

When a patient says, "I've had acupuncture before, and it didn't do anything," I'm always curious: was the issue point selection, or was it access? Were they being treated with a formula, or were they being met where their system actually was?

Why Acupuncture Changes as the Patient Changes

Patients sometimes expect acupuncture to be like a medication: you find the right prescription, and you repeat it. But the whole premise of acupuncture—at least as it has been practiced in the classical tradition—is that the body is not static. It's adaptive, and it's always responding to internal and external conditions. That means the "right treatment" is not a fixed object. It's a moving relationship.

A simple example: someone comes in with insomnia. The first few treatments might focus on settling the chest, easing the diaphragm, and reducing the internal revving that keeps them from dropping into sleep. They start sleeping better. Great. But then something interesting often happens: once the system isn't spending all night in fight-or-flight, other layers show up. Digestive sensitivity becomes easier to notice. Old grief appears. A long-standing shoulder tension becomes noticeable because the person finally has the bandwidth to feel it.

This can be unsettling for patients. "Why are we treating something new? I thought we were here for insomnia."

But it's not new. It was hidden under the louder pattern.

Regulation is not a straight line. When you shift one pattern, another pattern may become visible. That doesn't mean the treatment failed. It often means the system is reorganizing.

It also means that repeating the exact same points can become stale. A point that was essential in week one might be unnecessary in week six. A strong technique that was appropriate in an acute flare might be too much once the system is calmer. Conversely, once someone's reserves improve, you may be able to do more focused work on deeper patterns—scar tissue, longstanding joint restriction, chronic migraine circuits—that the system couldn't tolerate earlier.

A good clinician is always asking, "What is the body asking for now?" Not just *what did it ask for last time?*

This is one reason why "protocol acupuncture" often disappoints in chronic, complex conditions. Protocols assume sameness. Chronic illness is often defined by *instability and adaptation*—the system trying strategy after strategy to survive. You can't meet that with a rigid recipe and expect consistent results.

Why Results Depend on Physician Perception

This is a delicate topic because it can sound like arrogance: "Results depend on the physician." But it's not about ego. It's about perception—what the practitioner can notice, interpret, and respond to.

Acupuncture is a sensory medicine. The practitioner is reading:

- the patient's face and eyes,
- the quality of the voice,
- the way the breath moves,
- the texture and temperature of the skin,
- the tension patterns in the abdomen or neck,
- the pulse (when trained to do so),
- the immediate tissue response to needle insertion.

None of these pieces alone are magical. But together they create a live feedback system. The treatment is adjusted based on the response.

This is why two practitioners can treat the same diagnosis very differently, or why one gets consistent results, and the other doesn't. It's not always because one knows more theory. Sometimes it's because one is better at noticing what is actually happening in the room.

There's also a subtler piece: the practitioner's perception shapes the *intent* behind the needle. That word—intent—can make scientifically minded readers flinch. It shouldn't. Intent is simply the clinical hypothesis made tactile.

If I needle a point thinking, "I'm going to force this muscle to release," I tend to needle differently than if I'm thinking, "I'm going to invite this system to stop guarding." The second intent often produces a softer, more sustainable change—especially in patients with trauma histories or chronic pain sensitization. The needle becomes less of a crowbar and more of a tuning fork.

Patients pick up on this. Not consciously, necessarily. But their nervous system knows the difference between being managed and being listened to. And that difference affects the outcome.

This is also where humility matters. Perception is not infallible. A responsible practitioner is constantly testing their own impressions: *Did that point actually change the pulse? Did the tissue soften? Did the patient's breath deepen? Did their pain move or reduce?* If not, you don't blame the patient's "blocked energy." You reconsider your read.

Some of the best clinical moments are quiet ones: you place a needle, and something in the room drops—like a held note finally resolving. You can't manufacture that moment. But you can cultivate the conditions for it by paying attention.

The Limits of Acupuncture—and When It's Not Indicated

A chapter about regulation needs a section about limits, because regulation is not the same as omnipotence. Acupuncture can do a lot, but it does not replace emergency medicine, surgery, or the basic reality that some conditions progress despite good care.

There are several categories where acupuncture may not be appropriate—or may only be appropriate as support.

When there are red flags that need medical evaluation

If someone presents with symptoms suggestive of a serious condition—chest pain with exertion, sudden severe headache, neurological deficits, unexplained weight loss, fever of unknown origin, signs of infection, suspected fracture, bowel/bladder changes with back pain—acupuncture is not the first move. The first move is an appropriate medical evaluation.

A good acupuncture practitioner should be comfortable saying, "This is outside what I'm willing to treat without further workup." That's not defensive medicine. That's medicine.

When the body needs stabilization more than modulation

Some patients are so depleted, dysregulated, or medically complex that strong acupuncture techniques can destabilize them—at least initially. This includes some people with severe fatigue syndromes, active inflammatory flares, extreme anxiety states, or complex trauma presentations.

It doesn't mean acupuncture can't help. It means the approach needs to be gentler, slower, and often integrated with other supports. Sometimes the most skillful treatment is minimal needling—or none at all—paired with touch, breath work, lifestyle adjustments, or referral.

When the mechanism is structural in a way that needles can't fix

Acupuncture can reduce pain, improve function, and decrease guarding around structural problems. It can improve recovery after injury and surgery. But it cannot magically reconstruct a torn ligament, reverse severe joint degeneration, or remove a tumor.

It can help the system compensate more intelligently—and sometimes that's life-changing—but it shouldn't be sold as a substitute for appropriate orthopedic or oncologic care.

When there are clear contraindications or safety concerns

This is the unromantic part, but it matters:

- uncontrolled bleeding disorders or unsafe anticoagulation levels,
- severe needle phobia that overwhelms consent,
- local infection at the site,
- certain points, herbs, and techniques contraindicated with specific conditions
- inability to lie still or follow basic instructions (for safety),
- Inability to provide informed consent

Acupuncture is generally safe when practiced well, but "generally safe" is not the same as "always safe." A clinician who respects the limits is more trustworthy, not less.

When acupuncture becomes a way to avoid bigger decisions

This is harder to talk about, but it happens. Sometimes patients seek acupuncture because they want relief without confronting something else: an abusive work environment, a relationship that is breaking them down, untreated depression, a metabolic condition that requires significant lifestyle change, or a surgical issue they're afraid to face.

Acupuncture can support people through those decisions. It can reduce physiological noise, making clarity possible. But it shouldn't become a way to keep someone functional enough to stay in a situation that's actively harming them. Regulation is not meant to be sedation.

Dry Needling: An Ancient Technique Gone Modern

Dry needling is often framed as a contemporary, anatomy-based innovation: a clinician inserts needles into trigger points to relieve pain and improve function. Many physical therapists and sports medicine practitioners use it with real success, particularly in myofascial pain and movement-related complaints.

It's also, in a very real sense, acupuncture.

Not because of politics or licensing debates—those are separate conversations—but because the act itself is ancient. Needling tight, painful muscle bands is not a modern discovery. Classical physicians described "knots," "bindings," painful points, and needling strategies for them long before the language of trigger points existed.

What's modern is the framing.

Dry needling typically operates on a more localized model: treat the painful band, reset the muscle and improve movement. That can be exactly the right tool for certain cases—acute spasms, sports injuries, repetitive strain patterns—especially when combined with strength and mobility work.

Classical acupuncture, at its best, tends to embed local work inside a broader regulatory view. It asks additional questions:

- Why is that muscle tight in the first place?
- What is the global pattern of tone in the body?
- Is the nervous system in protection mode?
- Is there an internal driver—sleep loss, digestion, hormonal shifts, unresolved inflammation—that keeps reloading the tissue?

In other words, dry needling often excels at *changing the local tissue state*. Classical acupuncture aims to change the *state that keeps recreating the local problem*—while still respecting the local tissue.

Neither approach owns the truth. They simply emphasize different layers of the same body.

Where people get into trouble is when they assume that because dry needling can release a muscle, it's the whole story of needling. Or when acupuncture practitioners dismiss dry needling as crude, as if relieving a trigger point isn't real medicine. In the clinic, patients don't care about the ideology. They care whether they can turn their head without pain and whether the relief lasts.

A thoughtful integration looks like this: local needling when the tissue is clearly the limiting factor, and systemic regulation when the pattern is bigger than the tissue. Sometimes those happen in the same session. Sometimes they shouldn't.

One more point, because it's important: dry needling and acupuncture share tools but not educational or licensing standards. The deeper your needling—especially around the thorax, neck, and deep gluteal region—the more anatomy, safety, and clinical experience matter. "Ancient" does not mean "automatically safe." And "modern" does not mean "automatically precise." Skill does.

Regulation Is a Moving Target

If there's a single thread through this chapter, it's that acupuncture works best when we stop treating it like a substance and start treating it like a relationship.

The needle is a way of speaking to the body. Precision matters because the body is listening. Depth, angle, and timing are not pointless rituals; they're a way to communicate with an intelligent system. Locating a point is step one; getting it to respond is where the results happen. Treatments change because the patient changes—because a living system reorganizes when it's finally given a clean signal.

And the practitioner matters, not as a hero, but as an instrument. The clearer the perception, the cleaner the signal. The cleaner the signal, the more likely the body will do what it's been trying to do all along: adapt, stabilize, and return to a workable rhythm.

Acupuncture is not everything. It cannot replace imaging when imaging is needed. It cannot substitute for surgery when surgery is indicated. It cannot compensate for a life that is structurally unsustainable. But within its proper scope, it does something rare: it helps the body remember how to regulate itself without being coerced.

In the next chapters, we'll keep building on this idea—not by adding more techniques for the sake of it, but by refining what it means to think clinically in a system where the tool is never the point. The point is the change.

8

Herbal Medicine as Strategy

A common way people talk about Chinese herbal medicine—especially in the West—is as if it's an alternative pharmacy. You have symptom A, so you take herb B. Or you have diagnosis X, so you get formula Y. Sometimes that works well enough to convince someone the medicine is "real." More often, it fails in a predictable way: the herbs help a little, then stop helping; or they help one part and aggravate another; or they do nothing because the real problem isn't where the symptom is.

If you've been following the thread of this book, you already know why that way of thinking is incomplete. We're not treating isolated parts in a machine. We're working inside a living system that shifts with stress, sleep, food, hormones, seasons, trauma, infection history, workload, and a hundred other variables. That doesn't make it mystical. It makes it clinical. It means herbal medicine is not a fixed product—it's a strategy that gets revised as the system responds.

Herbal formulas, at their best, are like a well-designed plan: they anticipate resistance, they protect vulnerable terrain, they change the direction of a process rather than merely suppressing output. The "strategy" isn't abstract. It shows up in the selection of herbs, the ratios between them, the way they're prepared, and—most importantly—the way the prescription changes over time.

Let's unpack that. Not as theory for theory's sake, but as a way to see why Chinese herbal medicine can look confusing from the outside and yet be remarkably precise from the inside.

FORMULAS ARE DYNAMIC SYSTEMS, NOT FIXED PRESCRIPTIONS

A formula is not a list. It's an organized ecosystem.

If you read a typical herbal handout, it may look like a recipe: *Here are twelve herbs; boil them; drink.* That's not wrong, but it's like describing a symphony as "a lot of notes." The meaning is in the relationships—what's leading, what's supporting, what's restraining, what's harmonizing, what's preventing side effects, what's targeting a layer of physiology the others can't reach.

In practice, a formula behaves more like a dynamic system than a static prescription. It has:

- **A primary intention** (what change are we trying to produce?)
- **Secondary intentions** (what else must be addressed so the primary change is tolerated and sustained?)
- **Feedback sensitivity** (what will the body do in response, and how do we shape that response?)
- **Built-in constraints** (how do we prevent predictable complications?)

You can feel this difference when you watch formulas "move" a patient.

A purely symptomatic approach often produces a simple arc: symptom down, symptom up; relief, relapse. A strategic formula produces a different arc: symptom shifts location or character; energy changes; sleep adjusts; appetite responds; stool changes; emotional tone alters. Some changes feel like an improvement.

Others feel like the system reorganizing. The practitioner's job is to know which is which.

This is why it's so hard to judge herbal medicine from a single snapshot. If you evaluate the prescription as a fixed object—*twelve herbs for migraines*—you miss the point. You have to evaluate it as a step in a sequence: *what is the next best move in this system, today?*

That means two things that can be surprising:

1. **A good formula can be "wrong" next month.** Not because it failed, but because it succeeded and changed the terrain.
2. **A formula can be "right" even if it doesn't match the patient's diagnosis label.** Labels are coarse. Strategy is personal.

This is also why experienced herbalists often sound less certain than people expect. The certainty theater belongs to fixed prescriptions. A strategic clinician is watching a moving target—and adjusting with care.

THE HIDDEN ARCHITECTURE: HIERARCHY WITHIN FORMULAS

Classical herbalism does not pretend that all herbs in a formula are equal. A well-built prescription has an internal hierarchy. The traditional language for this is **chief, deputy, assistant, envoy**—a political metaphor that can feel outdated until you realize what it's pointing at: organization.

- The **chief** herb(s) sets the main direction—what the formula is primarily doing.
- The **deputy** herbs support the chief or address a major accompanying pattern.
- The **assistant** herbs do several possible jobs: they may reinforce, balance, prevent side effects, or address

secondary symptoms that would otherwise derail treatment.

- The **envoy** herbs guide the formula's action—sometimes toward a channel or region, sometimes toward a particular kind of movement (upward, downward, outward, inward), sometimes simply harmonizing the blend so it's tolerable.

This hierarchy is not just tradition. It's a way of thinking that prevents one of the most common clinical mistakes: treating everything at once with equal force.

Most complex patients have at least three stories happening simultaneously:

1. The **headline problem** (the symptom that brought them in).
2. The **background terrain** (the chronic pattern that makes the symptom possible).
3. The **adaptations** (the body's compensations—often protective—that come with their own costs).

If you try to "fix" all three with equal intensity, you either overwhelm the patient or cancel your own work. The hierarchy keeps you honest. It forces you to decide what is primary and what must be supported so the primary can change without harm.

Here's a simple example from the clinic.

A patient comes in with insomnia, palpitations, loose stools, and anxiety. A symptom-checklist approach might throw the kitchen sink at sleep: heavy sedatives, strong blood tonics, strong astringents. The patient sleeps for two nights, then feels foggy and more bloated, and the anxiety worsens. Why? Because the strategy didn't have an architecture. It treated "insomnia" like an isolated defect.

A hierarchical formula might instead prioritize **stabilizing the center** (digestion and fluid regulation), **settling agitation** without over-sedating, and **supporting blood** only to the extent it can be digested. The "sleep herbs" are present, but they're not the emperor.

The emperor is the strategy that makes sleep possible without collateral damage.

This kind of hierarchy is also why two formulas that share many ingredients can feel completely different in the body. The difference often lies not in the presence of a particular herb, but in its role and dose relative to the others.

WHY HERBS ARE COMBINED RATHER THAN ISOLATED

People ask this directly: "What's the herb for my problem?" It's a reasonable question if you grew up in a culture that treats medicine as single agents aimed at single targets.

Chinese herbalism answers, gently: *Your problem is not a single target.*

Herbs are combined for several pragmatic reasons, and none of them require mystical explanations.

1) To Create Direction Without Excess Force

Single herbs can be blunt instruments. That's not always bad—there are times we want blunt. But blunt tools come at a cost: they tend to create a strong movement in one direction while ignoring what that movement disrupts.

A formula can create direction with less violence. Think of steering a boat: you don't need an explosion; you need sustained, coordinated force.

A dispersing herb might be paired with something that protects fluids. A draining herb might be paired with something that supports digestion. A warming herb might be paired with something that prevents agitation. The goal isn't to "neutralize" the herb; it's to **shape** its effect so the body can actually use it.

2) To Treat the Pattern, Not Just the Symptom

Symptoms often sit at the end of a chain. The chain includes physiology, behavior, history, and sometimes months or years of adaptation. A single herb rarely addresses the chain.

Take chronic sinus congestion: the symptom is in the nose, but the pattern may involve digestion, fluid metabolism, immune reactivity, sleep, stress, and temperature regulation. A formula can address multiple links in that chain at once—gently enough that the system can reorganize.

3) To Address Layers

Many conditions are layered. A patient might have:

- underlying deficiency with
- secondary stagnation with
- episodic heat flares and
- a persistent damp component.

If you treat only the top flare, you chase symptoms. If you tonify only the deficiency, you may trap the stagnation. If you drain only damp, you may weaken the patient further.

A formula can be built to work across layers—sometimes sequentially within the same prescription, sometimes by setting the stage now for a deeper change later.

4) To Reduce Side Effects by Design, Not by Chance

Side effects in herbal medicine often come from predictable mismatches: too dispersing for someone depleted, too rich for someone with weak digestion, too descending for someone already prone to diarrhea, too warming for someone simmering under the surface.

In strategic herbalism, you don't wait for side effects and then apologize. You design around them.

That design is not conservative in the timid sense. It's conservative in the engineering sense: you assume stress points will be hit, so you build reinforcement into the structure.

5) Because the Body Responds to Relationships

This is subtle but important: the body often responds to combinations as combinations. Certain pairings are classic not because someone liked them, but because repeated observation showed that the effect is qualitatively different together than alone.

Sometimes the combination increases strength. Sometimes it changes the "texture" of the effect—making it smoother, slower, more targeted, less likely to overshoot. That texture matters in chronic illness, where overshooting is a common cause of regression.

TASTE, TEMPERATURE, AND DIRECTIONALITY: THE SENSORY LOGIC OF STRATEGY

One of the most underappreciated aspects of Chinese herbalism is how much it relies on **sensory categories**—taste, temperature, and movement—to describe what an herb does in the body.

To modern ears, that can sound pre-scientific. But in the clinic, it's often more useful than biochemical speculation. Not because biochemistry is irrelevant, but because we rarely have access to the full biochemical story of a living person with a unique history, diet, microbiome, nervous system calibration, and medication list. Sensory categories are a way of tracking reliable effects without pretending we can reduce the patient to a lab model.

Temperature: Warming and Cooling as Metabolic Instruction

When we say an herb is warming or cooling, we're not talking about the temperature of the tea. We're talking about the *kind* of change it induces.

- Warming substances tend to increase movement, circulation, digestive activity, and functional "spark." They can be profoundly stabilizing for someone cold, fatigued, or chronically constricted. They can also aggravate someone already running hot, inflamed, or agitated.
- Cooling substances tend to reduce inflammatory agitation, calm reactivity, and clear certain kinds of heat signs. They can be lifesaving in the right person and depleting in the wrong one.

The strategy isn't "warming good" or "cooling good." The strategy is: *What is the patient's system doing, and what kind of temperature instruction will move it toward stability?*

Taste: Not Flavor, Function

Taste in herbal medicine is not a culinary note. It's a shorthand for a function that shows up again and again in practice.

- **Acrid/pungent** tends to disperse and move—often outward or upward, often useful for constraint, stagnation, and certain surface-level problems.
- **Bitter** tends to drain, dry, or direct downward—often useful when there is heat, damp accumulation, or a need to "bring things down."
- **Sweet** tends to tonify, harmonize, and moderate—often useful for deficiency, tension patterns, and to protect the center from harsher herbs.
- **Sour** tends to astringe and stabilize—often useful for leakage patterns, excessive sweating, chronic diarrhea, or certain kinds of collapse.
- **Salty** tends to soften hardness and direct downward—often used for nodules, constipation patterns, or certain accumulations.

These are not rigid laws, and any experienced practitioner can name exceptions. But they're reliable enough that you can design a formula with them like an engineer uses material properties. You don't just ask, "Does this herb stop diarrhea?" You ask, "What is the mechanism of this diarrhea in this person, and what tastes and movements will correct it without creating a new problem?"

Directionality: Up, Down, In, Out—and the Geography of the Body

Directionality is where strategy becomes almost architectural.

Some herbs push outward—useful when something is trapped and needs venting. Some pull inward—useful when the system is leaking or scattered. Some lift—useful when clear yang doesn't rise, when there's sinking, prolapse, or chronic fatigue with heaviness. Some descend—useful when rebellion rises: nausea, hiccups, cough, anxiety that surges upward, headaches that feel like pressure climbing.

Directionality also relates to *where* in the body the formula is meant to act. Head vs. chest vs. abdomen vs. limbs; surface vs. interior; fluids vs. blood vs. qi dynamics.

This is one reason two people with a "cough" can need opposite formulas. In one, the problem is true rising rebellion with heat and irritability—descending and cooling makes sense. In another, the cough is due to dryness from fluids not ascending—warming and supporting ascent makes sense. Same symptom. Different directionality.

When formulas are built with taste, temperature, and directionality in mind, they stop being piles of herbs. They become maps.

WHY FORMULAS EVOLVE ACROSS VISITS (AND WHY THAT'S A SIGN OF COMPETENCE)

Patients sometimes worry when their prescription changes. They assume consistency equals correctness: *If you knew what was wrong, wouldn't you give me the same thing every time?*

That assumption makes sense if you believe treatment is a product. But if treatment is a strategy inside a changing system, then changing the formula is often the most rational thing you can do.

Here are a few concrete reasons formulas evolve.

1) Because the Pattern Has Actually Changed

This is the best-case scenario: the formula worked.

When a patient's sleep improves, their digestion shifts, their pulse changes, their tongue coat thins, their emotional reactivity softens—those are not side notes. They are the pattern-changing. The formula that matched the old pattern may now be too heavy, too drying, too warming, too dispersing, or simply no longer targeted.

Good treatment creates motion. Motion demands recalibration.

2) Because You're Treating in Phases

Many chronic conditions can't be solved in a single move without destabilizing the system.

You might first need to regulate digestion so that tonics can be absorbed. Or you might need to vent constraint so nourishment doesn't worsen pressure. Or you might need to clear a smoldering heat before you can safely warm and strengthen.

This phased approach can look inconsistent from the outside but feels coherent from the inside: each phase sets conditions for the next.

3) Because the Body Reveals Priorities Over Time

Some patterns are obvious at intake. Others only show themselves once the loudest symptom quiets down.

A patient comes in for migraines. You treat the migraine pattern, and it improves. Then their constipation becomes obvious.

Or their menstrual cycle shifts. Or their sleep becomes lighter and more dream-disturbed. Were those "new problems"? Sometimes. But often they were already present—just masked by the dominant complaint.

This is not failure. It's peeling an onion.

4) Because Dosage and Ratios Matter as Much as Ingredients

A formula can "change" without changing names.

Sometimes the exact same set of herbs is kept, but the ratio shifts dramatically. That can completely alter how the formula behaves: more emphasis on moving vs. building, more emphasis on clearing vs. harmonizing, more emphasis on drying vs. generating fluids.

This is why a competent herbalist can't be replaced by a formula database. The database can list ingredients. It can't think in ratios in the context of a real human being.

5) Because Life Happens Between Visits

This part is humbling, and it's where the clinic becomes a true laboratory.

Between visit one and visit two, a patient might get sick, travel, stop exercising, start a new medication, lose a job, reconcile with a parent, begin perimenopause symptoms, or develop new stress physiology. Sometimes the formula didn't "stop working." The conditions changed.

A strategy that doesn't adapt to life is not a strategy. It's a script.

SAFETY IS A FUNCTION OF KNOWLEDGE, NOT AVOIDANCE

There's a persistent myth that Chinese herbs are either "gentle and safe because they're natural" or "dangerous because they're unregulated." Both are half-truths that become unhelpful when they harden into identity.

Herbs are pharmacologically active substances. That's why they work. And because they work, they require knowledge.

Safety in herbal medicine is not achieved by avoiding strong herbs. It's achieved by understanding:

- what the herb does,
- when it's appropriate,
- what it tends to aggravate,
- how it interacts with the patient's constitution and medications,
- how preparation and dose change its character,
- and what signs tell you to adjust.

Strong Is Not the Same as Reckless

Some of the most useful herbs in classical practice are "strong" in the sense that they move blood, purge accumulation, transform phlegm, or clear intense heat. Avoiding them categorically would make the medicine toothless for serious conditions.

But using them without precision is irresponsible.

This is where experienced clinicians differ from dabblers: not in whether they use powerful tools, but in whether they can **forecast consequences**.

If you are going to use a strongly moving herb in someone with fragile sleep and anxiety, you build the formula so it moves without scattering. If you are going to clear heat in someone already dry, you protect fluids. If you are going to tonify someone prone to stagnation, you keep movement in the mix.

Safety is designed.

Preparation, Sourcing, and Dose Are Safety Issues

A conversation about herbal safety that ignores sourcing and preparation is incomplete.

- **Quality and identity** matter: correct species, correct part of the plant, correct processing.
- **Contaminants** matter: heavy metals, pesticides, adulterants—these are real-world risks that depend on supply chains.
- **Preparation** matters: decoction vs. powder vs. tincture changes extraction and effect. Traditional processing (like honey-frying, wine-processing, or steaming) changes tolerance and directionality.
- **Dose** matters: the difference between "supporting" and "overwhelming" is often not the herb but the amount.

A skilled herbalist thinks in these variables, not just the ingredient list.

Herb-Drug Interactions Are Real (And Manageable)

Another safety issue: interactions with pharmaceuticals.

Some herbs influence coagulation, blood pressure, liver enzymes, or neurotransmitter pathways. Many interactions are theoretical. Some are clinically significant. The point isn't fear. The point is coordination and transparency.

A good practitioner asks what you're taking, updates it each visit, and adjusts strategy accordingly. A good patient tells the truth, even if they worry they'll be judged.

SHARED RESPONSIBILITY: THE PHYSICIAN-PATIENT PARTNERSHIP IN HERBAL STRATEGY

Herbal medicine is unusual in modern healthcare because it places meaningful responsibility on the patient. Not because the patient is blamed if things go wrong, but because the patient is an active variable in the treatment.

If you're taking herbs at home, you are the one observing daily shifts. It's your job to be consistent in dosing and to notice how things move. A small change, like waking up with more energy, may be important feedback, even if your condition seems unrelated.

What the Physician Is Responsible For

A competent practitioner should:

- Make the strategy legible: *what are we trying to change, and how will we know it's changing?*
- Give clear instructions: preparation, dosing, timing, and what to do if you miss a dose.
- Screen for risk: pregnancy, anticoagulants, liver disease, complex medication regimens, allergies, prior reactions.
- Anticipate predictable reactions: when the patient might feel temporarily worse, what changes are acceptable, and what changes are warning signs.
- Create a feedback loop: a plan for follow-up, and a way to communicate if something unexpected happens.

If your practitioner hands you a bag of herbs with no plan and no follow-up, that's not the classical strategy. That's outsourcing.

What the Patient Is Responsible For

A patient doesn't need to become an herbalist. But they do need to participate.

That means:

- **Take the herbs as prescribed**—or say clearly when you can't. Many "herbs didn't work" stories are really "the plan wasn't feasible."
- **Report changes, not just whether the main symptom improved.** Energy, sleep, digestion, temperature, urination, mood, menstrual cycle—these are not side notes. They are the system talking back.

- **Disclose medications and supplements.** This isn't about permission. It's about safety and intelligent design.
- **Respect dose and duration.** Taking double because you want it faster, or stopping early because you feel better, both change the strategy.
- **Ask for clarity.** If you don't understand what the plan is, you're not being difficult—you're being responsible.

Shared responsibility also means shared humility. The practitioner is not omniscient. The patient is not passive. Both are observing the same weather system from different angles.

The Conversation That Prevents Most Problems

There's a simple question I ask patients, especially when we're using stronger formulas or when the case is complex:

"If something changes, how will you decide whether it's a good sign, a neutral sign, or a stop sign?"

That question forces the strategy into the open. It helps the patient feel oriented rather than anxious. It also disciplines the clinician to be explicit about what they expect. We talk through this question until we're both confident about our understanding.

We want change, and we don't want a patient to stop because the positive change makes them nervous. Some changes are acceptable—even desirable—because they indicate movement: a temporary change in bowel movements, a short-lived increase in urination, a brief surfacing of emotion, even a flare-up of the condition itself. Other changes are warning signs: allergic reactions, severe agitation, persistent nausea, worsening dizziness, unusual bleeding, rashes, or anything that feels sharply wrong. The changes we're concerned about, just like the herbs themselves, differ patient to patient.

When this conversation happens up front, herbal medicine becomes safer—not because nothing ever happens, but because when something does, the patient is prepared and it's handled intelligently.

STRATEGY IN THE REAL WORLD: A CASE-LIKE WALK THROUGH TIME

To make this concrete without turning the chapter into a textbook of formulas, let's walk through a familiar pattern in broad strokes.

A person comes in with chronic fatigue, "wired at night" insomnia, digestive fragility, and periodic anxiety. They've tried sedatives, magnesium and meditation. Sleep is still light. Their energy is inconsistent: they crash, then surge. They may have a history of overwork, long-term stress, maybe postpartum depletion, maybe years of pushing through.

A simplistic approach would label this "adrenal fatigue" and hand them tonics. Another simplistic approach would label it "anxiety" and hand them sedatives. Both can backfire.

A strategic approach might start by asking:

- Is the system unable to settle because it is **deficient** (not enough resources to change states)?
- Or because it is **constrained** (too much pressure, like driving with the parking brake on)?
- Or because digestion is failing and creating **phlegm/damp** that clouds and agitates?
- Or because there is a **heat** component—true heat or empty heat—from chronic strain?

The first formula might prioritize stabilizing the middle and settling agitation without heavy sedation. The second visit might reveal that once sleep improves slightly, the patient's digestion finally shows how weak it is—or that the anxiety was partly driven by stagnation and now emotion moves differently. The third visit might shift toward deeper nourishment, now that the center can handle it. Or it might pivot toward more movement because building too early creates pressure.

From the outside, this looks like inconsistency. From the inside, it looks like a clinician tracking the system's response and keeping the patient safe while moving them, step by step, into a different baseline.

That's strategy: not one clever formula, but a sequence of appropriate moves.

THE POINT OF ALL THIS: HERBAL MEDICINE AS CLINICAL THINKING

If you take one idea from this chapter, let it be this:

Herbal medicine is not the act of "taking herbs." It is the act of designing change in a complex human system—using herbs as adjustable instruments.

Formulas are dynamic systems. They have an architecture. Herbs are combined because bodies are complex and because combinations create direction, coverage, and restraint. Taste, temperature, and directionality are not quaint metaphors; they are practical ways of predicting how a substance will move a living process. Formulas evolve across visits because good treatment changes the terrain and because life changes the patient. Safety comes from knowledge—clear assessment, careful design, appropriate sourcing, dosing, and follow-up—not from avoiding anything powerful. And the entire process works best when responsibility is shared: the physician designs and monitors; the patient participates, observes, and communicates.

In other words, herbal medicine—done well—is not alternative. It's rigorous. It's responsive. It's honest about complexity. It's a strategy practiced one visit at a time.

In the next chapter, we'll take this same strategic lens and look at how a clinician decides what to prioritize when multiple patterns compete—because in real patients, they always do.

9

Constraint and Modern Life

If I had to name one pattern that quietly organizes modern illness—one pattern that shows up in digestive complaints, headaches, insomnia, menstrual problems, anxiety, chronic pain, autoimmune flares, fatigue syndromes, even "mystery symptoms" that don't fit neatly into a diagnosis—it would be constraint.

Not because people are weak, or sensitive, or failing to cope. But because the architecture of modern life is, in a very literal physiological sense, constraining.

We live in a world that asks for constant output without adequate completion. Constant attention without adequate digestion. Constant social signaling without adequate truth. Constant stimulation without adequate recovery. We ask the nervous system to perform sprint biology inside marathon conditions. And then we act surprised when the system starts to bind up.

Chinese medicine has always had language for this. You've already heard the idea that terms like stagnation and constraint are functional descriptions, not poetic metaphors. I won't restate that. What matters here is what happens when constraint becomes *normal*—when it's no longer an episodic response to a specific stressor, but the baseline shape of a person's physiology.

Constraint isn't a mood. It's a mechanical and regulatory state. And modern life is very good at producing it.

Why Constraint Is the Dominant Modern Pathology

In classical texts, constraint is often associated with the Liver—because the Liver's job is to keep things moving: qi, blood, emotions, digestion, menstrual flow, the smooth coordination of the body's internal timing. When that movement is blocked or forced into narrow channels, the whole system starts to compensate.

But if we reduce constraint to "Liver qi stagnation," we miss the point. Constraint is not limited to one organ system. It's a *relationship* between pressure and movement.

- Pressure is inevitable: responsibilities, uncertainty, change, grief, ambition, conflict.
- Movement is not guaranteed: time to process, space to breathe, permission to feel, the ability to act.

When pressure rises, and movement is allowed, the system adapts. When pressure rises, and movement is blocked—internally or externally—constraint forms. And once constraint forms, it tends to create more constraint. The body becomes less able to transition between states, less able to downshift, less able to complete cycles.

This is why constraint feels like being "stuck," but it's not just psychological. It's the autonomic nervous system stuck in readiness. The diaphragm not finishing its exhale. The jaw holding the sentence you didn't say. The gut tightening around the meal you ate too fast. The chest holding the grief you didn't have time for. The pelvic floor bracing against a day that never ends.

A person can be "high-functioning" and profoundly constrained. In fact, high-functioning is sometimes the most reliable mask.

Modern culture often treats stress as a mental problem. Think better, cope better, reframe, optimize. But stress is not primarily a thought problem. It's a mobilization state. It's chemistry and timing. It's cardiovascular tone, breath mechanics, inflammatory signaling, glucose regulation. It's whether the system can mobilize and then return.

Constraint is what happens when mobilization doesn't get to finish.

Emotional Regulation Is a Physiological Necessity (Not a Wellness Luxury)

There's a subtle cruelty in how we talk about emotions in health culture. Either emotions are treated as soft, optional, "mental health," separate from the body—or they're treated as moral obligations: regulate yourself, be calm, don't overreact.

In the clinic, you learn quickly that emotional regulation is neither a luxury nor a virtue. It's a physiological necessity. If the emotional system can't move, the body pays.

This isn't a poetic claim. It's observable.

Some patients get reflux when they swallow anger. Some get diarrhea when they anticipate conflict. Some get migraines after holding themselves together through a meeting. Some get insomnia not because they're "stressed," but because the body never got the signal that the danger is over. Some get menstrual clots after months of swallowing disappointment. Some develop chronic muscle pain because their nervous system cannot downshift without collapsing.

A useful question is not "Are you stressed?" Almost everyone is. A better question is: **Can your system complete a stress response?** Can it mobilize and then return? Can it feel something and then digest it? Can it be activated without becoming stuck?

In Chinese medicine terms, this is the difference between movement and constraint. In modern physiology terms, it's the difference between flexible autonomic regulation and chronic sympathetic dominance with impaired vagal recovery. Different language, same lived reality.

When emotional regulation fails, the body improvises. It builds workarounds:

- It tightens the muscles to create artificial containment.
- It shifts blood flow away from digestion.
- It increases heat to force movement.
- It dulls sensation to reduce input.
- It dissociates to survive.
- It develops symptoms that create boundaries the person cannot otherwise create.

Symptoms are often attempts at regulation.

That doesn't mean symptoms are "all in your head." It means the head and body were never separate to begin with.

The Emotional Map in Chinese Medicine: Not Psychology as Personality, but Psychology as Function

Chinese medicine has a different starting point from modern psychology. It's less interested in labeling personality and more interested in **how emotional states affect function**—and how functional states affect emotional capacity.

The classical model often describes "the seven emotions" (joy, anger, worry, pensiveness, sadness, fear, fright) not as a personality quiz, but as forces that move qi in predictable directions:

- Anger rises and disperses outward.
- Worry knots and binds.
- Fear descends.
- Sadness dissolves and depletes.
- Joy relaxes and opens—sometimes excessively.

These aren't moral judgments. They're movement descriptions.

You can also think in terms of the *shen* system—the constellation of mind-spirit functions distributed through the organs:

- **Shen (Heart)**: clarity, coherence, the sense of being here.

- **Hun (Liver)**: planning, vision, the capacity to move toward a future.
- **Po (Lung)**: sensation, grief, embodied presence, boundaries.
- **Yi (Spleen)**: thought, study, rumination, integration.
- **Zhi (Kidney)**: will, endurance, fear processing, deep reserves.

Again: not personality traits. Capacities.

When constraint becomes chronic, it tends to distort these capacities. A person might say, "I can't plan," "I can't focus," "I'm not myself," "I don't feel anything," "I can't stop thinking," "I'm exhausted but wired." These are not merely cognitive complaints. They are descriptions of systems losing flexibility.

In the clinic, you start seeing emotional patterns not as stories to interpret, but as *movement failures* to restore.

This is one reason Chinese medicine can be unexpectedly effective for conditions that sit awkwardly between "physical" and "mental." It doesn't require you to decide which side the problem is on. It treats the combined system.

Pressure Without Movement: How Constraint Turns into Heat, Pain, and Exhaustion

Constraint is not static. It has trajectories.

In the early phase, constraint looks like tightness, irritability, sighing, bloating, PMS, headaches, shallow breathing, variable appetite, sleep that feels "light," a sense of being on edge. The pulse may feel wiry. The tongue may still look fairly normal—some or all of these.

But the body doesn't tolerate blockage indefinitely. If pressure continues and movement doesn't return, the system begins to generate secondary patterns. This is where modern patients often live: not in pure constraint, but in constraint plus compensation.

Constraint generates heat

Pressure trapped in a closed system produces friction. In Chinese medicine, this is one of the simplest ways to understand how heat emerges—not only from infection or "inflammation," but from **stuck movement**.

Clinically, this heat might show up as:

- irritability that turns sharp
- insomnia with racing thoughts
- hot flashes or heat in the chest
- red eyes, dry mouth, bitter taste
- acne along the jawline
- urinary burning without infection
- flares of eczema
- a tongue that reddens at the sides or tip

It's common for patients to say, "I'm exhausted, but I run hot." That's not a paradox. It's a system burning fuel to force circulation through constraint.

Sometimes the heat is localized—temples, chest, throat, skin. Sometimes it becomes more systemic. And sometimes, over time, the heat begins to deplete fluids, creating dryness: dry eyes, dry stools, dry skin and a sense that the body is "running on fumes."

Constraint generates pain

Pain is often the body's most honest report: something is not moving.

The modern patient is full of pain patterns that look mechanical on imaging but behave like constraint in real life: neck and shoulder tension, jaw pain, rib-side tightness, pelvic pain, migraines, sciatica that flares with stress, and abdominal pain that appears with deadlines.

This isn't to deny structural issues. It's to notice that structure and regulation are entangled. Muscle tone is not just musculoskeletal—it's autonomic. Fascia is not just connective tissue—it's sensory, vascular, and reactive. Blood flow is not a constant—it's managed.

Constraint changes tone, perfusion and sensitivity.

One of the most consistent clinical experiences is this: a patient's pain improves not only when you "treat the area," but when you restore movement through the whole axis that feeds it—breath, digestion, sleep, emotional processing, circulation. Sometimes the "neck problem" is a diaphragm problem. Sometimes the "hip problem" is a boundary problem that the body is enforcing.

Physical injuries are one thing. Otherwise, chronic muscle pain is rarely the primary disease. If we can see what it says about the system, then the treatment can go far past the pain itself.

Constraint generates exhaustion

At first, constraint can look like high performance. The person pushes, the system mobilizes, adrenaline bridges the gap. They get through.

But chronic mobilization is expensive. It drains reserves. It disrupts sleep architecture. It impairs digestion. It increases inflammatory load. It destabilizes blood sugar. It creates a loop: fatigue → more effort → more mobilization → worse sleep → worse digestion → more fatigue.

In Chinese medicine, you often see this as a combined pattern: Liver constraint overacting on the Spleen, consuming qi; heat disturbing the Heart; the Kidneys asked to backfill the deficit. The person becomes simultaneously tense and depleted.

They will tell you, with a kind of confusion: "I'm tired all day and wired at night." Or: "If I stop, I crash." Or: "I can't relax—relaxing makes me anxious."

Those statements are not psychological quirks. They are descriptions of a system that no longer trusts downshifting because downshifting feels like collapse.

How Lifestyle Imprints on the Channels

It's tempting to talk about channels as abstract lines on a chart. In practice, channels are the lived interface between environment and physiology—where posture, breath, attention, and repetitive behavior leave marks.

Modern life is repetitive in very specific ways. It trains the body into constraint.

Consider a normal day:

- sitting with hips flexed and diaphragm restricted
- eyes locked at a fixed distance
- jaw subtly clenched in concentration
- shoulders protracted toward a screen
- breath held during cognitive effort
- notifications producing micro-surges of alertness
- meals eaten quickly or while working
- emotional tone managed to remain "professional"
- movement postponed until the end of the day—if at all

None of these are catastrophic. That's the problem. Constraint is rarely dramatic. It's cumulative.

Over months and years, the body adapts to the shape it's held in. The channels, as functional pathways, begin to show predictable patterns:

- **Gallbladder and Liver pathways**: lateral tension—temples, jaw, rib-side, IT band. The body's "decision and action" axis tightens when decisions are constant, and action is constrained.
- **Stomach and Spleen**: digestive timing breaks when meals are irregular, attention is split, and worry is chronic. The gut becomes the place where unprocessed experience collects.
- **Pericardium and Heart**: the chest becomes armored—emotional filtering becomes muscular tone.

Palpitations, chest tightness, shallow breath and sleep disturbances follow.

- **Lung and Large Intestine**: grief and boundary issues show up as skin problems, constipation, shallow breathing and immune fragility. The body cannot "let go" because it never got to finish processing.
- **Kidneys and Bladder**: deep reserves are drafted into daily functioning. The lower back tightens, the will becomes rigid, and fear becomes background noise.

Channels also reflect *timing*. When the circadian rhythm is repeatedly overridden—late-night screens, irregular sleep, travel, shift work—the body loses its internal sequencing. Treatment becomes harder not because the needles aren't right, but because the rhythm is not available to receive them.

This is why a patient can have "great treatment response" in the room and then lose it in three days. The clinic session is a brief return to movement; the lifestyle re-imposes the constraint.

The point isn't to blame lifestyle. The point is to make the mechanism visible. Once you see the imprinting, you can work with it.

Treating Stress Is Not the Same as Relaxation

One of the more unhelpful cultural ideas is that the solution to stress is relaxation.

Relaxation is a state. Moving between these states requires capacity.

Many constrained patients cannot relax—not because they refuse, but because relaxation feels unsafe. Their system equates downshift with vulnerability. Or with sadness that will finally surface. Or with the fear that if they stop, everything will fall apart.

So telling them to "relax" is like telling someone with a sprained ankle to "walk normally." It misunderstands the adaptation.

In the clinic, I'm often listening for a different question: **Can this person move between states?** Can they go up and come back down? Can they focus and then release focus? Can they feel anger and then return to baseline? Can they grieve without drowning? Can they rest without panic?

That is stress treatment.

Sometimes that looks calming, yes. Sometimes it looks like carefully releasing heat. Sometimes it looks like tonifying qi so the body doesn't have to clench to function. Sometimes it looks like moving blood, so the pain stops acting as a boundary. Sometimes it looks like *mobilizing* a depressed patient—not soothing them—because their constraint is frozen, not agitated.

Treating stress is not always about making someone feel comfortable in the moment. It's about restoring the system's ability to process pressure without locking.

This is also why some treatments "work" but don't last. If you only sedate the system—herbs that heavily anchor, points that only calm—the patient may feel better briefly and then rebound harder. They're not being restored; they're being managed.

There's a difference between a nervous system that is calm because it is regulated, and a nervous system that is quiet because it has been suppressed.

The first is resilient. The second is fragile.

The Physician's Job: Restore Movement, Not Provide Comfort

In the popular imagination, the ideal healer is comforting: warm hands, soothing voice, a treatment that feels like being wrapped in a blanket. Sometimes that's exactly what a patient needs, especially when there has been too much intensity for too long.

But comfort is not the goal. Movement is.

A good physician is not primarily a provider of relief. They are a restorer of circulation—in every sense of the word.

That includes:

- the circulation of blood and fluids
- the circulation of qi through the chest and diaphragm
- the circulation of digestion and elimination

- the circulation of sleep cycles
- the circulation of emotion through awareness and completion

Sometimes this restoration feels pleasant. Sometimes it feels like something finally unsticks—and that can be uncomfortable.

I've had patients cry on the table and apologize for it. I tell them the same thing: don't apologize. Things are moving.

Not every tear is healing, of course. But when tears come with a softening of the chest, a deeper breath, warmth returning to the hands, a pulse that unknots—those are signs of regulation returning. The body is doing something it couldn't do before.

Likewise, when a patient feels a surge of irritability after treatment, it's not always a bad sign. Sometimes it means the system is finding its mobilizing energy again—the energy that was previously trapped as tension or fatigue. The clinician's job is to guide that movement so it doesn't convert into heat or aggression, but into action, boundary, and appropriate change.

This requires a different kind of clinical maturity. You can't treat only what the patient wants ("make me calm") if what they need is to regain agency, or to metabolize grief, or to stop using their body as the place where unsaid things go.

The classics describe this as restoring the proper movement of qi. In modern language, you might say we are restoring regulatory range.

Either way, the work is not cosmetic.

Clinical Snapshots: Constraint Wearing Different Masks

Let me offer a few composites—real patterns, with identifying details blurred—not to "illustrate" theory, but to show how constraint hides in plain sight.

1) The productive insomniac

A woman in her forties, successful, reliable, the person everyone calls. She falls asleep fine, wakes at 2–3 a.m. and can't return to sleep. Her mind is not anxious exactly—just active, problem-solving. She's tired but functional. She has tight traps, jaw tension, occasional reflux, and cycles that have become shorter with more PMS.

This is not simply "stress." It's a system that mobilizes well and cannot downshift. The Liver is constrained, heat is beginning to rise, the Heart is disturbed, and the Spleen is taking collateral damage. If you only sedate her, you may get a few nights of sleep—and then the pattern returns.

Treatment has to restore the transition: discharge the stored mobilization, move the chest and diaphragm, cool without collapsing, support digestion so the body has enough qi to stop clenching, and make sleep a safe downshift again.

2) The frozen depressive

A man in his thirties, flat affect, low motivation, "not sad, just nothing." He sleeps too much but never feels rested. His digestion is slow, his stools are loose, and his limbs feel heavy. He has a history of prolonged stress that ended, but he never recovered. His pulse is not wiry; it's soft, possibly slippery.

This is constraint too—but it's constraint that has collapsed into dampness and depletion. If you treat him as anxious and try to calm him further, you can worsen the inertia. He may need gentle mobilization: warming and transforming damp, moving qi in a way that doesn't overwhelm, supporting the Spleen so there is enough upward lift for the spirit to return.

Stress didn't just rev him up. It shut him down.

3) The chronic pain patient with "normal tests"

A person with diffuse pain, fatigue, and a long list of normal labs. They've been told it's fibromyalgia, or central sensitization, or "nothing." They feel dismissed. Their body feels like it's bracing all the time. The pain moves. It changes with the weather, conflict, sleep, and meals.

Constraint is almost always part of this picture—not as a simplistic cause, but as a perpetuating mechanism. The body is guarding. The nervous system is scanning. The tissues are not receiving normal perfusion. The person is living in a state of unfinished threat response.

Treatment is often slow. The goal is not to chase pain around the body with local points. The goal is to rebuild trust in downshift: regulate the chest, support sleep, warm the center if needed, move blood if needed, address heat if present, and—crucially—help the patient recognize the early signs of constraint before it becomes a flare.

When Constraint Becomes Disease: The Systemic Spread

Constraint is rarely content to stay in one place.

This is one of the most clinically important realities in Chinese medicine: an unresolved pattern doesn't just persist. It *transforms*. It recruits other systems. It creates secondary damage.

A common progression looks like this:

1. **Qi constraint** (movement impaired)
2. **Heat** (friction, agitation, inflammatory tendency)
3. **Blood stasis** (microcirculatory impairment, fixed pain, clots, masses)
4. **Phlegm/damp** (metabolic and digestive consequences, brain fog, heaviness)
5. **Deficiency** (the cost of chronic compensation)

Not everyone follows this exact sequence. But the logic is consistent: blocked movement forces compensation; compensation has a price.

This is how you get the patient who started with "stress" and ended with:

- hypertension
- GERD that becomes chronic
- migraines that become weekly
- IBS that becomes inflammatory
- menstrual irregularity that becomes infertility
- skin flares that become autoimmune patterns
- anxiety that becomes panic
- insomnia that becomes depression
- fatigue that becomes collapse

To say "stress causes disease" is too vague to be helpful. The more useful statement is: **unresolved constraint becomes systemic because it disrupts regulation everywhere.**

In Chinese medicine, the Liver's smooth movement is not a luxury feature. It is a coordinating function. When it fails, the digestive system loses rhythm, the chest loses openness, the blood loses free flow, the spirit loses residence.

And once the spirit loses residence—once sleep is broken, once the Heart cannot settle—the body starts to behave like it is under threat even when it isn't. The person becomes a closed circuit.

The Modern Trap: Constant Activation Without Completion

One of the reasons constraint is so dominant now is that modern stressors are rarely resolvable in the way the body expects.

The stress response evolved for events with endings: run, fight, freeze, then return. But modern threats are often:

- social (status, conflict, evaluation)
- symbolic (emails, news, finances)
- chronic (caregiving, debt, unstable work)
- ambiguous (uncertain future, diffuse risk)

There is no clear moment when the tiger leaves.

So the body stays mobilized. And because the body can't stay mobilized forever, it does what it always does: it adapts. It builds a chronic pattern. Constraint becomes the new normal.

This is why the people who "handle stress well" are sometimes the ones who break later. They didn't handle stress; they *stored it.* They converted it into tension, heat, blood pressure, migraines, gut dysfunction and insomnia. They were praised for functioning while the bill accumulated.

What Restored Movement Actually Looks Like

If you're reading this as a patient, you might be wondering what any of this means practically. If constraint is so pervasive, what changes it?

The answer is not a single trick. But there are consistent themes in what works—both in treatment and in life.

1) Movement must be real, not conceptual

Insight helps, but the body needs physical completion: breath that reaches the lower ribs, walking that swings the arms, heat that vents through sweat, tears that arrive and end with catharsis, tremors that discharge tension after fear (yes, humans do this too when allowed).

Sometimes, acupuncture is the first place a person experiences this kind of completion in years: a spontaneous deep breath, a softening of the belly, warmth returning to cold hands, a sense of the mind settling not because it was forced, but because the body finally moved.

2) Regulation is built through rhythm

Constraint thrives in irregularity—late nights, skipped meals, constant switching, no transitions. Rhythm doesn't need to be perfect to be medicinal. It needs to be *reliable enough* that the body can predict a downshift.

This is why simple practices—consistent breakfast, a brief walk after lunch, dimming lights at night, a wind-down routine—can matter as much as sophisticated interventions. They aren't wellness trends. They're regulatory signals.

3) Boundaries are physiological

Some patients improve only when they start saying no. Not because no is empowering as a slogan, but because the body stops having to enforce boundaries through symptoms.

A migraine can be a boundary. So can IBS. So can insomnia. So can pelvic pain.

When a person can set a boundary directly, the body often doesn't need to do it indirectly.

This is not always possible in the short term—people have jobs, families, real constraints. But even small boundary restorations can change physiology: a protected lunch break, one evening without email, a conversation not postponed for another month.

4) Treatment targets movement, not just symptom suppression

Acupuncture points that move the chest and diaphragm, regulate the Liver and Spleen relationship, clear constrained heat, nourish fluids, and anchor the Heart can be transformative—but only when chosen based on the person's pattern, not the diagnosis on paper.

Herbal formulas that course and release may be appropriate early; later, the person may need to protect yin, move blood, or strengthen the middle so movement can occur without strain. The treatment evolves because the constraint evolves.

The most common mistake is to treat constraint as a static entity. It's not. It is a dynamic state that changes as soon as it changes—if that makes sense. When the first layer opens, you often discover what it was protecting.

A Quiet Reframe: Constraint Is Not the Enemy

One of the deeper clinical lessons is that constraint is not simply pathology. It is also protection.

A constrained system is trying to prevent something: collapse, overwhelm, conflict, loss or exposure. It is a strategy that once worked.

So the goal is not to "break" constraint. The goal is to make it unnecessary.

When patients feel that you're trying to take away their armor, they resist—and they should. When they feel that you're helping them build real capacity underneath it, the armor softens on its own.

This is where Chinese medicine, at its best, feels less like force and more like persuasion. You are not imposing health. You are restoring the conditions in which health is the body's default.

Where This Leaves Us

Constraint is not a niche concept. It is one of the main ways modern life becomes illness—and one of the main ways illness becomes chronic.

If you can learn to recognize constraint early—before it converts into heat, before it hardens into pain, before it drains into exhaustion—you can change trajectories that otherwise look inevitable.

And if you're a practitioner, this chapter is an invitation to treat stress with more seriousness than "calming." The work is not to comfort the patient into tolerating their life. The work is to restore movement so that life becomes metabolizable again.

In the next chapter, we'll take this further into the question that inevitably follows: once movement returns, what exactly is moving? Not just qi in the abstract, but the deeper substances—blood, fluids, essence—and the rhythms that keep a person coherent over time.

10

Reproduction, Reserve, and Timing

Reproductive medicine attracts certainty-seeking. Understandably. When someone wants a child—or wants to *not* want a child anymore, and can't—the question becomes urgent in a way that few health concerns do. The body becomes a clock, a test strip, a number on a lab report, a countdown. People who would normally tolerate ambiguity suddenly find themselves bargaining with it.

Chinese Medicine doesn't remove that urgency. It just refuses to reduce fertility to a single switch you can flip.

In the classical view, reproduction is not a separate department of the body. It is a high-level function that sits downstream of many ordinary choices: nourishment, rest, repair, emotional load, illness history, work patterns, aging. It depends on *reserve*—and reserve depends on how the whole system has been living.

This chapter is about that reserve. Not as a mystical substance, and not as a moral judgment ("you should have taken better care of yourself"). Reserve is simply the body's stored capacity to build, repair, and reproduce without breaking its own rhythm. And reproduction, more than almost anything else, is a timing question: *Do you have enough, at the right moment, in the right place, for long enough?*

We'll talk about Blood and Essence as foundations, cycles as expressions of reserve, why preparation often matters more than intervention, how to support reproductive health without promising outcomes, and why modern life so reliably injures the very reserves reproduction depends on.

I'll reference earlier ideas lightly where they belong—things like stress physiology, rhythm instability, and how patterns show up in the body—but I won't re-teach them here. This chapter needs its own depth.

BLOOD AND ESSENCE: THE FERTILITY FOUNDATIONS

In biomedicine, fertility is often framed through hormones, anatomy, and timing: AMH, FSH, estradiol, luteal progesterone, follicle counts, tubal patency, semen parameters. Those matter. I read those labs. I'm not allergic to them.

But in the classical Chinese frame, fertility is built on two foundational resources:

- **Blood**: not just red fluid, but the body's capacity to nourish, moisten, and provide material support to tissues and functions.
- **Essence (Jing)**: not a metaphor for "vitality," but a way of describing deep constitutional capacity—developmental, reproductive, and regenerative potential.

If you want a grounded translation: Blood is what the body can *spend* to build and maintain tissues. Essence is what the body can *invest* from its deeper savings account when it needs growth, development, or reproduction.

Why this distinction matters clinically

People often come in wanting to "balance hormones." Sometimes they've been told their problem is estrogen dominance, low progesterone, PCOS, endometriosis, or unexplained infertility. They want a lever.

Chinese Medicine is often more interested in a different question: **What resource is missing—or what resource is being burned too fast—that makes hormone signaling unstable?** Hormones are messengers. They don't deliver a message into an empty room and expect a pregnancy to assemble itself. The room needs materials.

Blood and Essence are those materials.

When Blood is insufficient or poorly mobilized, you see it in the reproductive landscape: thin endometrial lining, dry cervical fluid, erratic ovulation patterns, delayed recovery after miscarriage, fatigue that lingers beyond what "normal labs" can explain. It can also show up as anxiety that feels wired-but-tired because Blood also anchors the mind. (You've likely seen this connection in real life: when your reserves are low, everything feels louder.)

When Essence is depleted, the signature is deeper: long-standing reproductive difficulty, repeated early losses, premature ovarian insufficiency patterns, low sperm count with poor motility and morphology, developmental or endocrine fragility that precedes the fertility story. Essence deficiency can also appear after prolonged illness, chronic inflammation, chemo, or years of overextension that never really allowed recovery.

This is not about blaming anyone for having "low essence." It's about acknowledging something modern medicine often sidesteps in practice: **biology has limits, and those limits are shaped by time.**

The classical map: Kidneys, Tian Gui, Chong, and Ren

Classical texts locate reproductive capacity in the **Kidneys**, not because the kidneys-as-organs make babies, but because the Kidney system in Chinese Medicine governs Essence, development, maturation, and the capacity to hold and anchor life processes.

You'll also see the term **Tian Gui**—often translated as "Heavenly Water"—which is essentially the maturation signal that enables reproductive function. When Tian Gui arrives, puberty happens. When it declines, menopause approaches. In between is the reproductive window, which is not identical to the modern fertility window but overlaps with it.

Two extraordinary vessels are central here:

- **Chong Mai** (Penetrating Vessel): often described as the "Sea of Blood," involved in deep regulation of blood and reproductive function.
- **Ren Mai** (Conception Vessel): involved in nourishment, gestation, and the yin aspect of reproductive capacity.

When these networks are well supplied—by Blood and Essence—and the body's regulatory function is coherent, reproductive physiology tends to be robust. When supply is low or regulation is disrupted, reproduction becomes fragile.

This is the first important pivot: **infertility is not a single organ problem.** It's a whole-body resource and timing problem that expresses itself through the reproductive system.

The male side of the equation (often neglected)

Classical texts discuss reproduction in a way that includes men, but modern fertility culture often makes fertility a woman's burden until proven otherwise. Clinically, that's not just unfair—it wastes time.

In Chinese Medicine terms, male fertility depends heavily on Kidney Essence as well, but it also depends on:

- Blood's ability to nourish tissues and maintain healthy fluids
- Liver function in the sense of smooth movement and regulation (stress, constraint, heat)
- Spleen function in the sense of transformation and resource generation (metabolic robustness)

Men with high stress, poor sleep, heavy alcohol, heat exposure (saunas, hot tubs, laptops), chronic inflammation, or long-standing overwork can show classic signs of diminished reserve—sometimes even when their testosterone looks "fine."

And because sperm production cycles take time, interventions are never instantaneous. The body doesn't respond to panic. It responds to conditions.

CYCLES ARE EXPRESSIONS OF RESERVE

Most people think of reproductive cycles as calendars: a period every month, ovulation around day 14, luteal phase, repeat. Or, in fertility tracking: LH surge, BBT shift, cervical fluid peak.

That's useful. But it's incomplete.

In Chinese Medicine, a cycle is not just a repeating event—it's a **pattern of resource allocation**. A cycle tells you how the body spends, replenishes, and holds reserve over time.

If the reserve is strong, the cycle tends to be resilient. If the reserve is weak, the cycle becomes a negotiation.

The deeper idea: rhythm as evidence of capacity

Earlier, we discussed the body's need to maintain dynamic relationships—activity and rest, heat and cooling, tension and release. Cycles are where that relational intelligence becomes visible.

A reproductive cycle asks the body to do something expensive:

- Build tissue (endometrium)
- Mature a follicle and ovulate
- Create and maintain a luteal environment
- Either shed and reset, or sustain a pregnancy

Each step requires coordinated signaling and adequate material support. If you don't have enough Blood, the endometrium may be thin or unstable. If you don't have enough Essence, follicular development may be inconsistent, or the system may not tolerate the metabolic cost of sustained progesterone production. If stress mobilizes the system into chronic vigilance, the body may choose survival priorities over reproduction—quietly, without drama, until you try to conceive.

This is not the body being "broken." It's the body being conservative.

Cycles are not only monthly

When I say cycles, I don't only mean menstruation. I mean:

- **Daily cycles**: energy upon waking, appetite rhythms, afternoon crashes, evening second winds
- **Seasonal cycles**: winter storage vs summer dispersion, how recovery changes across the year
- **Life-stage cycles**: puberty, postpartum, perimenopause, aging
- **Stress cycles**: repeated activation without resolution

Reproductive capacity sits inside all of that. A person can have a "normal period" and still have poor reserve signals elsewhere: poor recovery from exertion, chronic cold hands and feet, frequent illness, insomnia that doesn't track with sleep hygiene, libido that feels disconnected from the body.

Conversely, someone can have irregular cycles but excellent reserve—if the irregularity is driven by a specific, reversible constraint rather than depletion. That distinction matters. It changes the whole plan.

What reserve looks like in the clinic (without making it mystical)

Reserve is not a single symptom. It's a *texture*.

In someone with a strong reserve, you often see:

- Good recovery after exertion or stress

- Stable appetite and digestion (not perfect, but coherent)
- Sleep that repairs, even if it's not long
- Skin and hair that reflect nourishment
- Emotion that moves and settles rather than looping
- A cycle that adapts to travel, stress, or mild illness without falling apart

In someone with low reserve, you often see:

- Recovery that takes too long
- Symptoms that flare with small stressors
- The feeling of "running on adrenaline"
- More pronounced sensitivity to temperature, stimulants, skipped meals
- A cycle that is easily disrupted by the very life that person is living

None of this is a moral assessment. It's a clinical reading.

And it helps answer one of the most practical questions in fertility care: **Is the next step to push for function, or to rebuild capacity first?**

PREPARATION OVER INTERVENTION

There's a certain kind of fertility care that feels like forcing a locked door: more stimulation, more supplements, more tracking, more protocols. Sometimes that's necessary. Sometimes it's lifesaving. But often, especially in chronic or unexplained cases, forcing function without preparation creates a pattern: short-term movement, long-term fragility.

Chinese Medicine is at its best when it plays the longer game.

Preparation doesn't mean passivity. It means choosing steps that make the body better able to sustain what you are asking it to do.

Why the "quick fix" instinct backfires

When someone has been trying to conceive for a year (or five), every month becomes a referendum. They want something that *changes the outcome this cycle*. The practitioner feels that pressure too. It's easy to start treating the calendar instead of the person.

But if the underlying issue is low reserve, chronic inflammation, constraint, or dysregulation, then "making ovulation happen" isn't the same as creating a pregnancy that can implant and hold.

The classical approach often looks like this:

1. **Stabilize the terrain** (sleep quality, stress physiology, digestion, circulation, inflammation signals)
2. **Build the resources** (Blood, Essence, fluids)
3. **Regulate the movement** (smooth function, appropriate warmth, appropriate cooling, appropriate containment)
4. **Then support the reproductive event** (ovulation, luteal support, implantation environment)

This sequence isn't dogma. It's pragmatic. If you try to build a house during an earthquake, you don't need better nails. You need the ground to stop moving.

"But I'm 38. I don't have time."

I hear this constantly, and it's real. Preparation cannot become an excuse for indefinite delay. Chinese Medicine must respect time pressure, especially with age-related decline in ovarian reserve.

So how do we reconcile preparation with urgency?

By being specific about what preparation means and how long it should take.

Some preparation is slow by nature—building Blood after years of depletion, restoring endocrine resilience after chronic stress, and improving sperm parameters. But some preparation is surprisingly quick: reducing inflammatory load, improving sleep depth, shifting nervous system tone, supporting digestion so nutrients become available, and resolving stagnation patterns that interfere with pelvic circulation.

A realistic clinical stance is:

- **We prepare and intervene at the same time**, but we do it intelligently.
- We don't pretend we can manufacture reserve overnight.
- We look for early signals that the body is becoming more coherent.

Preparation is not waiting. It's building conditions.

The preconception window: what we actually do

People ask for "fertility acupuncture" as if it's a standardized product. In reality, preconception care is a set of decisions based on pattern differentiation.

What we're often doing, clinically, is some combination of:

- **Nourishing Blood**: improving tissue building and anchoring capacity
- **Supporting Kidney Essence**: enhancing deep reserves and reproductive robustness
- **Regulating Liver movement**: reducing constraint that disrupts cycles, ovulation quality, and pelvic circulation
- **Strengthening Spleen function**: ensuring nutrition becomes a usable resource rather than dampness, fatigue, or inflammation.
- **Clearing heat or damp-heat** where inflammation and irritation are part of the terrain
- **Calming and settling the mind** so the body can shift out of chronic vigilance

These aren't abstract categories. They show up as concrete

changes: more stable energy, less premenstrual reactivity, better cervical fluid, more consistent basal temperatures, fewer inflammatory flares, improved sleep depth, reduced pain, improved libido and a body that feels less like it's being dragged through the month.

Notice what I did not say: "We guarantee pregnancy."

We prepare the body to be a better host for pregnancy. That is meaningful, whether or not conception happens on schedule.

The overlooked part of preparation: learning the body's language

One of the most important roles of preconception care is teaching someone to recognize the difference between:

- effort that builds reserve

and

- effort that spends reserve

Many high-functioning people have been rewarded for overriding. They can push through fatigue, ignore hunger, work late, train hard, travel often, run on coffee, and still look "fine." Fertility is often where that strategy stops working.

Preparation involves a kind of re-education: not in the form of scolding, but in the form of feedback. The body responds. The cycle responds. Symptoms respond. The question becomes: *Can you hear it?*

SUPPORTING REPRODUCTIVE HEALTH WITHOUT GUARANTEES

If you do fertility work long enough, you learn to speak carefully.

Not because you're afraid of being wrong, but because the stakes are tender. People don't just want a baby. They want the grief to stop. They want their body to stop betraying them. They want a story that makes sense.

Chinese Medicine can offer coherence. It cannot offer certainty. No medicine can.

What we can promise—and what we can't

We can often promise:

- careful observation
- a plan that matches the person, not the label
- regular reassessment based on response
- support for sleep, mood, digestion, pain, inflammation, and resilience
- improved cycle quality and reduced symptom burden
- a partnership that includes referrals and integration with biomedical or other professional care when appropriate

We cannot promise:

- conception by a deadline
- avoidance of miscarriage
- that age, genetics, anatomy, or severe pathology will yield to herbs and needles

This is not pessimism. It's an ethical reality.

In practice, the most compassionate thing you can do is to **separate worth from outcome**. People internalize infertility as personal failure. They interpret every intervention as a test of whether their body is "good enough." A clinician's job is to keep the frame clean: we are working with physiology, timing, and probability —not virtue.

Fertility is probabilistic, even when everything looks good

Even in ideal conditions, conception is not guaranteed each cycle. The body is not a vending machine. It is a living system responding to thousands of variables, many of which we can't measure well.

This is where Chinese Medicine can be psychologically stabilizing—not by offering magical control, but by offering a different relationship to uncertainty: *We strengthen the conditions. We improve the odds. We pay attention. We adjust.*

That stance is surprisingly relieving for many patients, especially those exhausted by the constant binary of "pregnant/not pregnant."

Working alongside modern reproductive medicine

Some people come to Chinese Medicine after IVF fails. Others come before they start. Some do both in parallel. I'm not interested in ideological purity. I'm interested in outcomes and integrity.

The key is to understand what each system is good at:

- Biomedical reproductive medicine is excellent at **structural assessment, hormonal manipulation, and procedural support**—especially when specific barriers are identified (tubal obstruction, severe male factor, anovulation not responding to lifestyle changes).
- Chinese Medicine is often excellent at **improving systemic conditions** that influence egg quality, sperm quality, implantation environment, inflammation, stress physiology, and recovery from procedures.

In a well-integrated plan, Chinese Medicine can support:

- preparation before retrieval or transfer
- recovery after stimulation (sleep, digestion, mood, inflammation)
- pelvic circulation and tissue nourishment
- reducing side effects and supporting resilience through the process

But integration requires honesty. If someone has severely diminished ovarian reserve at 43, we may still work to support their health and their process—but we don't pretend herbs can reverse time. If someone has blocked tubes, we don't "move qi" and call it done. We help them make clear decisions.

The clinical art: choosing the right entry point

A line from earlier in the book matters here: *The clinical art is choosing an entry point that is safe, effective, and responsive—and then watching what changes.*

In fertility work, that principle becomes even more important because people have limited time, limited money, and limited emotional bandwidth.

Sometimes the entry point is very direct: regulate the cycle, support ovulation, address luteal insufficiency patterns, clear damp-heat. Other times, the entry point is indirect: restore appetite, improve sleep depth, reduce constraint, rebuild after years of depletion. The right entry point is often the one that changes the system fastest—because it restores the body's own intelligence.

And yes, the right entry point can shift over time. Fertility care is not a linear protocol. It's a series of course corrections.

When it doesn't work: holding grief without abandoning reason

One of the hardest parts of fertility care is sitting with outcomes that don't match effort. People do everything "right" and still don't conceive. Or they conceive and lose the pregnancy. Or they make embryos and none implant. Or they stop treatment because it becomes too much.

In those moments, Chinese Medicine should not become a consolation prize or a spiritual bypass. It should remain what it is: a medicine that supports life.

Sometimes the work becomes about:

- restoring the body after loss or procedures
- helping someone sleep again
- rebuilding appetite, warmth, steadiness
- supporting the relationship that has been strained by the process
- helping someone find their next decision without coercion

This is still medicine. It's not the outcome they wanted, but it is not nothing.

MODERN REPRODUCTIVE STRESS: HOW RESERVES GET INJURED

If you want to understand why fertility struggles are so common now, you don't need a single villain. You need a systems view.

Modern life injures reserves in predictable ways. Not just through "stress," but through specific patterns of depletion, inflammation, and dysregulation that accumulate over years.

1) Chronic sympathetic tone: living in "on"

Earlier, we explored how chronic activation shows up in the body—tension patterns, rhythm disruption, the sense of being unable to land in rest fully. In fertility, chronic sympathetic tone matters because reproduction is not an emergency function. It's a long-term investment.

When the body perceives a threat—whether emotional, financial, relational, or physiological—it reallocates resources. It prioritizes survival, vigilance, and short-term coping.

This can look like:

- ovulation that becomes inconsistent under pressure
- luteal phases that shorten in high-stress months
- libido that disappears not because of hormones, but because of the nervous system state

- inflammation that becomes more reactive

People often hate hearing this because it sounds like: "Just relax." That's not what I'm saying. Most people cannot relax on command, and telling them to do so only adds pressure.

The clinical question is different: **What allows your system to shift into repair mode, reliably, without forcing it?** That's where real fertility support begins.

2) Under-eating and over-training: the fashionable injury

A surprising number of fertility cases involve some version of "not enough." Not enough calories, not enough carbs, not enough rest days, not enough fat, not enough recovery between workouts, not enough warmth in the system.

This is not always an eating disorder. Often it's disguised as wellness:

- disciplined meal plans that quietly underfeed
- high-intensity training layered on top of demanding work
- stimulant use to override fatigue
- fear of weight gain that keeps the body in scarcity

From a Chinese Medicine perspective, chronic scarcity injures Blood and Essence. From a biomedical perspective, it can suppress GnRH signaling, alter thyroid conversion, disrupt leptin and insulin signaling, and elevate cortisol. Different languages, same lived outcome: the body does not feel resourced enough to reproduce.

And here's the part people don't want to hear: you can be strong, accomplished, and "healthy" by many modern metrics—and still be running a major deficit.

3) Inflammation as background noise

Inflammation doesn't always feel like an acute illness. Often it's a low-grade, persistent terrain: skin issues, gut reactivity, brain fog, joint stiffness, frequent infections, or pelvic inflammation.

In Chinese Medicine, this may show up as heat, damp-heat, phlegm, toxin patterns—again, not as mystical categories, but as shorthand for observed clusters: irritation, swelling, thick fluids, stickiness, reactivity, and poor clearance.

Inflammation matters for fertility because implantation is a delicate immunological event. So is sperm function. So is egg quality. A chronically inflamed terrain can be subtly hostile to reproduction.

This is one reason "unexplained infertility" often isn't truly unexplained—it's just that the standard workup isn't built to describe terrain well.

4) Sleep debt and circadian confusion (and why it's not just about hours)

We've already discussed sleep rhythm instability earlier in the book, so I won't rehash it. But I will say this: fertility care without sleep repair is usually limited.

Not because sleep is a moral virtue, but because it is when the body does a significant portion of its repair and endocrine recalibration. If sleep is shallow, fragmented, or delayed night after night, the body's capacity to build Blood and protect Essence weakens. People can compensate for a while—until they can't.

5) The mental load: invisible work that drains reserve

One of the most modern fertility stressors is not physical at all. It's the constant cognitive and emotional overhead:

- decision fatigue
- long-term uncertainty

- hypervigilance about timing, symptoms, test results
- relational strain
- the quiet grief of "life not happening on schedule"

This mental load has physiological effects. It changes breathing, digestion, temperature regulation, muscle tone, and hormonal signaling. It changes how the body allocates resources.

In the clinic, I often see the turning point not when someone "gets the right herb," but when their life no longer feels like a perpetual test.

That can mean therapy. It can mean changing jobs. It can mean saying no to a family dynamic. It can mean stopping tracking for a month. It can mean choosing IVF—or choosing to stop. The correct choice is not universal. The correct choice is the one that reduces the chronic stress on the system.

6) Delayed childbearing and the collision with biology

This is a sensitive topic because it sits right where cultural pressure lives. People delay childbearing for good reasons: education, finances, career, partnership timing, healing from trauma, caring for family, and simply not being ready. These are not errors.

And biology still matters.

In Chinese Medicine terms, Essence naturally declines with age. In biomedical terms, oocyte quality and quantity decline, and the risk of miscarriage rises. We can support resilience through that transition. We cannot negotiate with time indefinitely.

The most grounded fertility conversations are the ones that respect both truths:

- You are not wrong for living your life.
- Your body may still have limits that require different strategies and expectations.

When a clinician can hold that without blame, patients often feel something rare: relief mixed with clarity.

TIMING: WHEN THE BODY IS READY (AND WHEN IT ISN'T)

Chinese Medicine is sometimes caricatured as slow. In fertility work, it's more accurate to say it's **timing-oriented**.

We're not only asking, "What pattern is this?" We're asking, "What time is it in this person's physiology?"

Two people can have the same diagnosis—PCOS, endometriosis, recurrent miscarriage—and require entirely different strategies because their timing is different:

- One has robust reserves but poor regulation (needs smoothing, clearing and mobilizing).
- One has poor reserves and fragile stability (needs building, anchoring, warming, conserving).
- One has a mixed picture: stagnation on top, deficiency underneath (very common).

Timing also matters across the month, even if we're not doing a rigid "phase-based protocol." The body doesn't do the same thing in the follicular phase as it does in the luteal phase. Our treatments should respect that.

But the deeper question of timing is this: Is your body in a season of building or **a season of spending?**

If it's spending—through overwork, stress, inflammation, inadequate nourishment—then fertility interventions often feel like pouring water into a bucket with a hole. The answer isn't always to stop everything. Sometimes that's impossible. The answer is to patch the hole as much as you realistically can and then choose interventions that don't worsen the leak.

A CLINICAL CLOSING: WHAT THIS FRAME OFFERS

If you take nothing else from this chapter, take this:

- Reproduction relies on **reserves**.
- The reserves are built from **Blood and Essence**, and expressed through **cycles**.
- The most effective fertility care often emphasizes **preparation**, not because we avoid intervention, but because intervention works better in a prepared system.
- Ethical care supports reproductive health **without guaranteeing outcomes**.
- Modern life reliably injures reserve, not through a single cause, but through chronic patterns that keep the body from repairing.

Chinese Medicine is sometimes sold as an alternative to modern fertility care. I don't find that framing helpful. What it truly offers is a different center of gravity: away from panic and toward conditions. Away from obsession with a single number and toward the whole terrain. Away from heroic forcing and toward intelligent support.

That doesn't make the path easy. It makes it more coherent.

And for many people, coherence is the first form of hope that doesn't collapse under pressure.

In the next chapter, we'll look at how this same concept of reserve—and the body's relationship to timing—shows up in aging, chronic illness, and recovery: the long arc where medicine becomes less about fixing and more about stewardship.

11

Digestion as the Central Axis

People love the phrase *you are what you eat* because it sounds clean and controllable. If food is the input and the body is the machine, then the solution is simple: choose better input.

But in the clinic, that idea breaks down fast.

Two people eat the same meal. One feels steady and clear. The other gets bloated, anxious, sleepy, foggy, or inflamed. Another does everything "right"—organic, gluten-free, low sugar, high protein, no seed oils—and still can't tolerate breakfast without nausea or fatigue. Someone else lives on noodles and late-night snacks and somehow holds together.

So we have to refine the slogan.

You are not what you eat.

You are what you can *transform*.

It's now what's in the food.

It's what you can get *out of* the food.

That word—*transformation*—sits at the center of Chinese Medicine. Not as a metaphor. As clinical instruction. The question is never just "what are you consuming?" It's "what is your system capable of doing with what you consume?" And when that capacity falters, the downstream effects are not limited to the gut. They show up as energy problems, blood problems, mood problems, immune problems, menstrual problems, sleep problems—often long before a lab value waves a flag.

Earlier, we talked about the body as a communicating network, and about chronic illness beginning as functional drift before it becomes structural damage. Digestion is one of the first places that drift becomes visible—not because digestion is weak, but because digestion is *central.* It sits at the crossroads where environment becomes body.

This chapter is about that crossroads: why the middle of the body—literally and physiologically—governs far more than appetite and bowel movements, and why rebuilding digestive function is often the most direct way to restore global regulation without fighting the body symptom by symptom.

"YOU ARE WHAT YOU EAT" IS INCOMPLETE

When patients tell me, "I'm eating so clean," I usually believe them. The problem is that "clean" is not a physiological category. The body does not recognize moral purity in food. It recognizes temperature, texture, timing, volume, and complexity. It recognizes stress chemistry during meals. It recognizes whether you chew. It recognizes whether your nervous system is braced or receptive. It recognizes whether you're eating at 11 p.m. under blue light after three hours of scrolling. It recognizes whether your digestive fire is strong enough to cook what you're throwing into the pot.

In classical terms, food and drink enter the Stomach, to be "rotted and ripened" (a vivid phrase), then the Spleen extracts what can be used and sends it upward to become Qi and Blood. The rest is sent downward and out. That description is old, but it's not mystical. It's an observation-based model of a very practical reality:

- **If transformation is strong**, the body can tolerate variation.

- **If transformation is weak**, even "good" food becomes a burden.

THIS IS why diet advice so often fails. It assumes the digestive capacity is stable. But in many cases, the digestive capacity is the variable. The same meal that nourishes you in one season of life becomes hard to process in another. The same high-fiber "gut health" protocol that helps one person wrecks another because their system can't generate enough warmth, secretion, and motility to handle it.

And once transformation weakens, people start reacting to food as if it were the enemy. They cut more, restrict more and rotate more. They become afraid of meals. They become detectives of ingredients instead of students of their own physiology.

Sometimes avoidance is appropriate. But it's not a strategy for building health. It's a strategy for reducing friction.

Health, in the classical view, is not fragility. It doesn't need everything to be perfect. It's resilience—your capacity to receive, transform, distribute, and eliminate. Digestion is where that resilience is trained daily.

TRANSFORMATION IS THE CORE OF HEALTH

In Chinese Medicine, the Spleen and Stomach are not just organs. They are a functional axis—what we often call the *Middle Burner*. Think of it as the body's processing plant.

What does a processing plant do?

1. It breaks down raw materials.

2. It sorts what's useful from what's not.

3. It distributes resources to where they're needed.

4. It manages waste so it doesn't clog the system.

That is digestion. But it's also immunity. It's also metabolism. It's also the stability of thought. It's also the quality of blood. It's also whether fluid moves or congeals. It's also whether you wake up with usable energy or wake up already behind.

This is why classical doctors paid such close attention to appetite, taste, stool quality, abdominal temperature, morning energy, and the feeling after eating. These are not "gut symptoms." They're indicators of how well the body is converting life into living tissue and usable fuel.

When that conversion is strong, other systems have room to regulate themselves. When it's weak, everything else starts compensating. The Liver pushes. The Heart overworks. The Kidneys dip into reserves. The Lungs lose their crisp descending function. Symptoms scatter. People get a list of diagnoses instead of a coherent picture.

There's a temptation—especially in modern settings—to treat the scatter directly:

- reflux with acid blockers,
- constipation with stimulants,
- diarrhea with binders,
- fatigue with caffeine and willpower,
- anxiety with sedatives,
- inflammation with suppressants.

Sometimes those tools are necessary. I'm not arguing against them. I'm arguing against the *habit* of seeing symptoms as independent enemies. In classical reasoning, the more symptoms you have, the more likely it is that the core function—transformation and distribution—is compromised.

If you rebuild that function, symptoms often reorganize on their own. Not because the body is magical, but because the network has regained a reliable center.

DIGESTION GOVERNS ENERGY, BLOOD, AND THOUGHT

In Western physiology, we're used to separating categories: digestion is gastrointestinal; energy is mitochondrial; mood is neurotransmitters; cognition is brain. Those are useful distinctions for research. They're less useful for clinical coherence.

Classical medicine insists—again, by observation—that these domains are not separable in lived experience. The Spleen and Stomach are central because they produce the postnatal Qi that powers daily life. They are also the source of Blood, which anchors the mind and nourishes tissues. And the Spleen is directly linked to a kind of thinking: *Yi*—the mind's capacity to hold, study, concentrate, and digest experience.

That last line can sound poetic until you see it in people.

Energy: the feeling of having "fuel"

There's a specific kind of fatigue that comes from Middle Burner weakness. It isn't just low energy—it's low *availability*. People describe it like this:

- "I can do things, but I can't sustain them."
- "I crash after meals."
- "My energy feels ungrounded—like it flickers."
- "If I skip a meal, I unravel."
- "Mornings are heavy; afternoons are worse."

This fatigue often comes with a body that feels puffy, heavy, or damp; or with a mind that feels thick, as if thoughts have to push through fog. From a classical lens, that's not "laziness" or even "adrenal fatigue." It's a sign that the system isn't extracting clean, usable Qi from food and fluids—and that the byproducts of poor transformation (what we call Dampness and Phlegm) are accumulating and obstructing clear movement.

Blood: not just a substance, but a stability

When digestion is steady, blood is replenished steadily. When digestion falters, blood deficiency can develop—not always dramatically, not always on labs, but functionally.

Patients don't come in saying, "I'm blood deficient." They say:

- "My sleep is light and restless."
- "My hair is thinning."
- "I get palpitations when I'm tired."
- "My periods are lighter and shorter, or I spot."
- "My anxiety is worse when I'm hungry."

From a classical view, the Heart houses the mind, but the mind needs Blood as its material anchor. A person with weak digestion may generate enough stimulation to keep going—caffeine, stress hormones, adrenaline—but not enough Blood to feel settled. They can appear "fine" and still feel internally unmoored.

This is why so many chronic cases have a pattern that looks like this:

1. digestive weakness,
2. then fatigue and brain fog,

3. then sleep and mood instability,

4. then diffuse inflammation, pain, or hormonal irregularity.

It's not a rigid sequence, but it's common enough that you start listening for it as a story—a pattern.

Thought: when the mind can't digest

The Spleen's relationship to thought is one of the most clinically useful—and most misunderstood—ideas in Chinese medicine.

It does **not** mean "the Spleen causes anxiety."

It means something subtler: when the Middle Burner is weak, *thinking becomes less efficient and more sticky*. The mind chews without swallowing.

People can't finish a thought. Or they can't stop thinking the same thought. They ruminate, worry, over-prepare, over-research, and overanalyze. They become mentally busy but internally unnourished.

And the loop tightens:

- Weak digestion → less clear Qi and Blood → thought becomes sticky

- Sticky thought → more worry and sympathetic tone → digestion becomes weaker

A clinician learns to hear this loop in the way someone speaks: the long lists, the inability to prioritize, the sense of being overwhelmed by small decisions. Often, these are not personality traits. They are physiological states. Much of what we think of as personality traits is like this.

WARMTH AND RHYTHM: THE MIDDLE DOESN'T LIKE SURPRISES

If I had to reduce digestive health to two words in classical terms, they would be **warmth** and **rhythm**.

Not because everyone should eat hot soup forever. Not because cold food is evil. But because transformation requires a stable inner climate and predictable timing.

Warmth: the fire under the pot

The classics state that the Spleen likes warmth and dryness and dislikes cold and dampness. Modern readers sometimes interpret that as superstition. But clinically, it's easy to verify.

A person with robust digestion can tolerate cold smoothies, iced drinks, raw salads. A person with weak digestion often cannot. They may crave those things—especially if they run hot or inflamed—but they pay for them later with bloating, loose stools, fatigue, or a heavy head.

This isn't about rules. It's about capacity.

Cold constricts. It slows. It reduces enzymatic and motility efficiency. It requires the body to spend extra energy just to bring the contents to functional temperature. If the system is already low on warmth—what we call Spleen Yang deficiency—then cold becomes not just a preference but a stressor.

A useful clinical image is this: digestion is like cooking. If the flame is strong, you can add ingredients, and the pot keeps simmering. If the flame is weak, every new ingredient drops the temperature, and the stew never truly cooks. It just sits—fermenting, producing gas, heaviness, and residue.

Rhythm: timing is a medicine

Rhythm is the other half of digestive strength. The Middle Burner is not designed for constant grazing, constant stimulation, or irregular timing. It likes a pattern it can anticipate.

People often underestimate this because they think digestion is purely mechanical: food in, nutrients out. But digestion is a coordinated sequence of secretion, motility, bile flow, microbial signaling, and nervous system state. Coordination improves with predictability.

In the clinic, it's striking how often a case improves not because we found the perfect food, but because we re-established a basic rhythm:

- eating earlier in the day,
- not skipping breakfast if it destabilizes them,
- leaving space between dinner and sleep,
- reducing late-night snacking that mimics stress relief.

You can call this circadian biology. Classical medicine would call it aligning with the natural timing of Qi movement. Either way, the lived outcome is the same: when rhythm returns, symptoms lose intensity.

Warmth and rhythm are not dietary ideology

It's important to say this plainly: "warm" and "rhythmic" do not mean rigid. They mean *appropriate*. A strong person can bend without breaking. A weak person needs steadiness long enough to rebuild. The goal is not to become someone who can only eat at 7:12 p.m. The goal is to restore the kind of digestive confidence that allows flexibility again.

That's how you know function is rebuilding: the world stops feeling like a minefield of triggers.

EXCESS INFORMATION CAN HARM THE SPLEEN

There's an old teaching: the Spleen is harmed by *pensiveness*—excess rumination, worry, overthinking. In modern life, that teaching has become almost painfully literal.

We usually talk about diet as food. But what is your mind eating all day?

A patient will say, "My digestion is sensitive," and then casually describe a routine that includes:

- waking up and immediately checking messages,
- working while eating,
- listening to podcasts while driving,
- scrolling in the bathroom,
- eating dinner with the news in the background,
- falling asleep to a glowing screen.

That is not rest. That is not rhythm. That is a nervous system trained to be alert through every meal, and a mind trained to never finish processing.

From a classical perspective, that constant intake creates a form of Dampness—an accumulation of unprocessed material. Not just in the gut, but in the mind. The Spleen's job is to transform and transport; if input never stops, transformation never completes.

Clinically, this shows up in a particular pattern:

- appetite that's present but easily disrupted,
- bloating that tracks with stress more than food,

- alternating stool patterns,
- brain fog that worsens with mental effort,
- a feeling of "I can't hold things"—memory, focus, even emotional boundaries.

This is why some people's digestion improves when they change nothing about their macros and everything about their attention. When they eat without working. When they stop feeding themselves information while feeding themselves food. When they let the body do one thing at a time.

You don't need to make a religion out of mindful eating. But you do need to recognize that digestion is not a side task. It is a whole-body state.

If the Spleen is the axis of transformation, then attention is one of its fuels.

EATING AS PARTICIPATION IN THE ENVIRONMENT

One of the most grounding aspects of classical medicine is its refusal to imagine the body as separate from its world.

Food is not just nutrients. Food is climate, season, soil, storage, culture, and relationship. It carries the imprint of place. It carries the imprint of how it was prepared and eaten.

To say "you are what you eat" is still too narrow. A truer statement would be:

You are what you do repeatedly, taken as broadly as possible.

Season and place are part of digestion.

The classics emphasize seasonal eating not as lifestyle fashion, but because the body's needs shift with climate. In winter, warmth and storage are emphasized. In summer, dispersion and cooling are emphasized. Transitional seasons strain the Middle Burner more easily—dampness rises, appetite becomes inconsistent, and heaviness appears.

In practice, this means that the same person may digest very differently in August than in January. It also means that dietary advice lifted from one climate and applied to another can be quietly destabilizing. A raw, cooling diet may feel "healthy" in theory, but erode digestive warmth over time in a cold, damp environment.

Again: this is not ideology. It's an observation.

Cooking is a form of medicine

Cooking is not just flavor. It is pre-digestion.

For someone with robust digestion, raw foods can be enlivening. For someone rebuilding, cooking often becomes a key therapeutic step—not because raw food is bad, but because the body doesn't have to spend as much effort warming and breaking it down. The meal arrives already partially transformed.

This is also why soups, stews, congees, and simple warm breakfasts have such a consistent place in traditional healing cultures across the world. It's not nostalgia. It's physiology.

Eating is relational

There's also a social aspect that modern nutrition rarely touches.

People digest better when they feel safe. They digest better when meals are not rushed, hidden, or riddled with guilt. They digest better when eating is not an argument with themselves.

Some of the most dramatic digestive improvements I've seen came when a patient stopped trying to "win" against their body. They started feeding themselves like someone worth caring for. They simplified. They stopped performing health. They began participating in their own life again.

The Middle Burner, in classical terms, is the pivot between Heaven and Earth—between what comes in and what becomes you. Eating is one of the few times each day when that pivot is explicit. If you treat it as an interruption, the body often follows your lead.

DIGESTIVE WEAKNESS AS THE QUIET ROOT OF CHRONIC DISEASE

Not every chronic illness starts in the gut. But digestive weakness is one of the most common *maintaining factors* in chronic illness—especially when the case includes fatigue, inflammation, dysregulation, and sensitivity.

You can think of it this way: chronic disease often involves a reduced margin of adaptability. Digestion is where adaptability is replenished daily. If the replenishment system is weak, the margin continues to shrink.

This is one reason chronic cases can feel like they "spread." First, it's mild IBS. Then it's fatigue. Then it's anxiety. Then it's a hormonal irregularity. Then it's skin rashes. Then it's joint pain. Then it's food reactions. Then it's chemical sensitivity. The person feels like they're becoming allergic to life.

From a classical view, that spread is not random. It's what happens when the center cannot govern distribution and clearing.

Dampness and Phlegm: when transformation leaves residue

Poor transformation doesn't just fail to produce enough usable Qi and Blood; it also produces residue. Classical medicine calls that residue Dampness and Phlegm—again, not as pathology labels, but as descriptions of behavior:

- Dampness is heavy, lingering, turbid, and obstructive.
- Phlegm is more consolidated, more mobile, and can lodge anywhere—joints, chest, sinuses, even the mind.

In modern terms, you might think of inflammatory byproducts, metabolic congestion, poor clearance, dysregulated fluids, microbiome shifts, and neuroinflammation. The classical language is broader because it's pattern-based rather than mechanism-based.

But the clinical observation is consistent: when the Middle Burner is weak, the body tends to accumulate what it cannot process.

This is why chronic bloating is rarely just "gas." It's often a sign of systemic processing trouble. And why chronic phlegm, sinus congestion, cysts, swollen lymph nodes, and mental fog can all share a digestive root even when the person's primary complaint is nowhere near the stomach.

A clinical pattern you'll recognize

A common chronic case looks like this:

- The person had stress, overwork and irregular meals for years.
- They had mild digestive signs—bloating, loose stools, reflux and cravings.
- Then their system got suddenly taxed (infection, pregnancy, surgery, grief, burnout).
- After that, their baseline never returned.

Now they have a diagnosis—maybe several—but the felt experience is: "My system can't recover."

When we treat these cases only at the branch—only at the most dramatic symptom—we often miss the quieter truth: they no longer have a reliable center. Their energy production is inconsistent. Their blood building is compromised. Their clearing pathways are congested. Their thoughts are sticky. Their sleep isn't restorative.

Rebuilding the Middle Burner doesn't solve everything overnight. But it gives the case a stable axis. It sets up the system for improvement.

Why modern suppression can backfire (even when it helps)

This is delicate territory because many medications are life-changing and appropriate. But it's also true that symptom suppression can sometimes deepen the underlying weakness if we mistake relief for resolution.

Consider three common examples:

- **Chronic acid suppression** can reduce pain and protect tissue, but it can also reduce the digestive signaling that helps transform food, especially in people already prone to cold and weakness.

- **Chronic laxative use** can create dependency and further weaken motility and fluid regulation.

- **Constant antimicrobial approaches** (whether herbs, supplements, or repeated "cleanses") can sometimes strip the terrain without rebuilding function, leaving the person more sensitive over time.

The issue is not "medicine is bad." The issue is strategy. Are we rebuilding capacity, or are we managing consequences?

Classical medicine is often at its best when it does both—protects the branch while rebuilding the root—without pretending that relief equals repair.

REBUILDING FUNCTION RATHER THAN SUPPRESSING SYMPTOMS

If digestion is the axis, then treatment is often less about attacking a diagnosis and more about restoring the conditions under which transformation can happen again.

That sounds gentle. It isn't always. Rebuilding function can require uncomfortable honesty about pace, habits, and the difference between stimulation and nourishment.

The first move is usually not "more supplements"

When digestion is weak, people often respond by adding complexity: enzymes, probiotics, binders, bitters, adaptogens, nootropics, electrolytes, shakes, powders, and protocols stacked on protocols.

Sometimes those help. Often, they overwhelm.

A weak Middle Burner tends to do poorly with constant novelty. It does better with a period of simplification—fewer ingredients, fewer meal variables, fewer changing inputs—so the clinician and the patient can observe what is actually happening.

In classical terms, we're protecting the Spleen's ability to transform by reducing its burden. Remember, it's not what is in the food or supplement, it's what you can get out of it.

Rebuilding warmth is often foundational

If signs point toward cold in the middle—loose stools, undigested food, fatigue after eating, preference for warmth, bloating relieved by heat—then rebuilding warmth becomes central. This may involve:

- warmer cooking methods,
- reducing iced and raw intake for a time,
- using aromatic, warming herbs that move and awaken the Middle,
- supporting the body's Yang without over-stimulating it.

There's nuance here. Many chronically inflamed people *feel hot* and assume they need more cooling foods. But sometimes the heat they feel is not robust warmth—it's "floating heat," agitation, or inflammatory friction sitting on top of weak digestion. In those cases, indiscriminate cooling can worsen the root weakness and leave the person colder, foggier, and more inflamed over time.

The clinician's job is to tell the difference, not to follow a protocol.

Rhythm is a treatment, not a lifestyle tip

Rebuilding rhythm is often more powerful than people expect. Not perfection—just reliability.

A common turning point is when someone stops eating late at night. Not because late eating is morally wrong, but because the body cannot both digest and descend into deep rest. If digestion stays active into the night, sleep becomes lighter; if sleep is lighter, digestion is weaker the next day. The loop continues.

Another turning point is when someone stops skipping meals as a form of control. Fasting can be useful for some constitutions and patterns. For others—especially those with blood deficiency, anxiety, irregular cycles, or post-illness depletion—skipping meals can destabilize the system and intensify reactivity.

Again: the point is not a doctrine. The point is matching rhythm to physiology.

You rebuild by making the Middle Burner feel safe

This is a phrase I use with patients: *we're going to make your digestion feel safe again.*

Safe means:

- meals that are predictable enough to build trust,
- portions that don't overwhelm,
- an emotional environment that isn't rushed or combative,

- fewer “tests” and more consistency.

When the Middle feels safe, appetite becomes more honest. Cravings become less urgent. The body stops swinging between extremes—overeating and under-eating, diarrhea and constipation, hyperfocus and brain fog.

This is also where the earlier point about information matters. A person can eat the perfect meal and still not digest it if their nervous system is in fight-or-flight, their mind is flooded, and their attention is fractured.

Sometimes the most medical thing you can do is eat without input. Twenty minutes. No phone. No news. Just one task. Let the system complete a cycle.

Clinical reality: progress is often quiet

When digestion improves, people sometimes miss it because the change isn’t dramatic.

They don’t wake up feeling like a new person. Instead, they notice small, reliable shifts:

- They’re hungry at normal times.
- They can eat and keep going without crashing.
- Their stool becomes formed and regular without force.
- Their limbs feel warmer.
- Their mind is less sticky.
- Their sleep deepens incrementally.
- Their skin calms.
- Their cycles stabilize.

- Their reactivity decreases.

These are not "gut outcomes." These are system outcomes. They tell you the axis is stabilizing.

Why this approach matters for chronic and complex cases

Chronic disease often tempts practitioners into chasing complexity: more testing, more targeting, more specialized interventions. Sometimes that's appropriate. But in many cases, complexity becomes a kind of avoidance—an attempt to bypass the slow work of rebuilding foundational function.

In classical practice, you learn to ask a simple, almost stubborn question:

Is this person generating enough usable Qi and Blood each day to sustain repair?

If the answer is no, then the most brilliant intervention will have limited traction. The body cannot be built with empty hands. And it cannot be cleared with clogged pathways.

Rebuilding digestion is not glamorous. It's often the work of weeks and months. But it changes the conditions under which everything else becomes possible.

THE MIDDLE AS A TEACHER

There's one more reason digestion deserves this central place: it teaches you how to think clinically.

The Middle Burner forces you to stop treating the body as a set of disconnected problems and start seeing it as a transformation economy: input, processing, distribution, storage, and waste. It forces you to attend to timing, temperature, and capacity—not just chemistry. It forces you to respect that symptoms can be intelligent signals from a system trying to adapt.

And it forces humility.

Because digestion is not fully under conscious control. You can't will peristalsis into being. You can't think your way into enzyme secretion. You can't biohack your way out of a nervous system that feels unsafe.

But you *can* create conditions that make regulation more likely.

That is the quiet genius of classical medicine: it is less interested in control than in cooperation. Not because it lacks power, but because it recognizes what chronic illness keeps trying to teach—health is not produced by force alone. It is produced by function. And function is produced by conditions.

In the next chapters, we'll build on this axis and look at how other systems—Liver movement, Heart stability, Lung descent, Kidney reserves—either support the Middle or destabilize it. But keep digestion as a reference point. If you ever feel lost in the complexity of symptoms, come back to the question that steadies the entire case:

What is this person able to transform—food, fluids, experience—into usable life?

When you can answer that clearly, the treatment path stops being a collection of tricks. It becomes a coherent strategy.

CHAPTER 12: PAIN AS OBSTRUCTION AND MESSAGE

Pain makes people honest.

Not morally—clinically. Pain has a way of stripping away the stories we tell ourselves about what we can tolerate, what we should ignore, what we can push through. It forces the nervous system to speak up. It reorganizes priorities. It changes posture, breath, sleep, mood, appetite, relationship. And it brings people into the clinic who have been "fine" for years—until they weren't.

The problem is that pain also makes people reactive. Patients want it gone yesterday. Practitioners want to fix it quickly, partly out of compassion and partly because no one likes to sit with a suffering person and say, "This will take time." Entire medical systems are designed around rapid suppression because it's measurable and marketable: pain score down, job done.

But Chinese medicine—at least in its older, clinically serious forms—doesn't treat pain as an enemy to be silenced. It treats pain as information about movement.

That doesn't mean we romanticize it. Pain is not "a teacher" in the motivational-poster sense. It's often brutal, limiting, and demoralizing. Some pain is dangerous and demands urgent care. Some pain is senseless—injury, degeneration, based on damage. And some pain persists long after tissues have technically "healed," because the nervous system has changed its rules.

Still, pain is rarely random. It has shape. It has timing. It has a relationship with rest, weather, stress, digestion, sleep, menstrual cycles, breathing and fear. It has patterns.

If you can read those patterns, pain becomes less mysterious—and less tyrannical. Not because you've learned a trick, but because you've learned what it's pointing to.

This chapter is about that: pain as a failure of movement, pain as obstruction, pain as a message. And what it means to treat pain without becoming trapped by it.

PAIN IS OFTEN A FAILURE OF MOVEMENT —NOT A THING IN ITSELF

A common modern framing is: pain equals tissue damage. If something hurts, something must be broken.

That's sometimes true. A fracture hurts for a reason. Appendicitis hurts for a reason. An infection hurts for a reason. There are pains you do not negotiate with.

But a surprising amount of pain—especially musculoskeletal pain, headache patterns, pelvic pain, many types of neuropathic pain—doesn't correlate cleanly with tissue damage. People have terrible MRIs and no pain, and "normal" imaging with debilitating pain. Even when damage exists, it often doesn't explain the full intensity or persistence.

Classical Chinese medicine starts from a different assumption: pain is frequently what happens when normal movement is interrupted.

Movement here doesn't just mean joint range of motion. It means the ability of a region, a tissue, or a system to do its job without strain: to circulate, to warm and cool appropriately, to repair, to adapt, to transition from tension to relaxation and back again.

When movement is reduced, the body doesn't merely lose function. It becomes louder. The nervous system increases surveillance. Local tissues become sensitive. Muscles brace. Breathing changes. The area becomes precious and guarded. And pain becomes a kind of protective alarm—sometimes appropriate, sometimes excessive.

In older language, you'll hear, "Where there is obstruction, there is pain. Where there is free flow, there is no pain." That line gets repeated so often it can feel like a slogan. The deeper value is this: it invites you to look for *what is not moving*.

- Is the joint itself mechanically restricted?
- Is the fascia stiff, densified, protective?
- Is blood flow cold, ischemic or slow to recover?
- Is fluid movement swelling, edema or inflammatory congestion?
- Is nerve function inflamed, irritated or hypersensitive?
- Is the person trapped in bracing, unable to exhale, unable to soften?

Pain often lives at the boundary between what the body is asking for and what the person is forcing.

One of the most useful clinical questions I know is deceptively simple: **What movement is being prevented—locally or systemically?**

Sometimes it's literal. A frozen shoulder hurts because the capsule has tightened and the brain has learned to protect it. A neck that can't rotate hurts because the surrounding tissues have become vigilant. A pelvic floor that can't release hurts because the body has decided that release is unsafe.

Sometimes it's less literal. Someone with migraines that come every Sunday night might not have "a head problem" at all. They might have a week-long buildup of sympathetic drive and poor eating, followed by a sudden drop in adrenaline and a rebound vascular and inflammatory response. The pain is the endpoint of a weekly rhythm that's become pathological.

In that sense, pain is not a thing you treat. It's a relationship you change.

ACUTE PAIN AND CHRONIC PAIN ARE NOT THE SAME PROBLEM

If you treat all pain the same way, you'll either under-treat danger or over-treat adaptation.

In the clinic, I separate pain into two broad categories—not because life is that tidy, but because decision-making improves when you respect the difference:

Acute pain: the alarm that matches the moment

Acute pain is often tied to a recent event: injury, infection, surgical trauma, sudden inflammation, a clear flare of arthritis, a kidney stone, a disc protrusion or an acute nerve irritation.

The key features are:

- It has a relatively clear onset.
- It changes rapidly.
- It often responds to appropriate rest and protection.
- It often comes with signs of active tissue threat: heat, swelling, sharpness, redness, fever and night pain that's new and escalating.

In Chinese medicine terms, acute pain often involves more obvious excess: sudden obstruction, heat, swelling and spasm. The body is mobilizing resources, and the system is loud.

The goal here is not heroic. It is intelligent containment: calm the acute threat, keep the person safe, prevent maladaptive guarding from becoming the new normal, and support recovery. You don't want to "power through" acute pain, but you also don't want to freeze a person into immobility for weeks unless that's truly necessary.

This is where good triage matters. Some acute pain needs imaging, labs and emergency care. Chinese medicine is not a substitute for that. A clinician who treats severe new pain as "just stagnation" is not practicing medicine—they're practicing denial.

Chronic pain: the alarm that has rewritten the rules

Chronic pain is different. It may begin acutely but persist beyond the expected tissue healing time. Or it may creep in gradually, woven into years of posture, stress, sleep debt, inflammation, and micro-injuries.

Chronic pain tends to have:

- A history of flare and remission.
- Triggers that include stress, weather, fatigue, certain foods and poor sleep.
- A strong relationship to mood, attention, and fear (not because it's "in the mind," but because the nervous system is involved).
- A pattern of compensation: one area hurts, then another takes over and starts hurting too.

In Chinese medicine terms, chronic pain is rarely a single excess. It's often a layered pattern: obstruction plus deficiency, stagnation plus weakness, local congestion plus systemic inability to resolve it. The loudness of pain can coexist with low reserves.

This is where simplistic approaches backfire—especially approaches that chase the loudest symptom. We've already talked earlier in the book about how over-clearing or over-warming can create second- and third-order problems. Chronic pain is one of the places that matters most.

In chronic pain, the goal is not simply to "turn pain off." The goal is to change the conditions that keep pain necessary.

That takes time. And it requires a different kind of therapeutic relationship—one that treats the patient as an adaptive organism, not a broken machine.

WHEN YOU SUPPRESS PAIN TOO SUCCESSFULLY, YOU LOSE THE MAP

Pain has a reputation for being useless. People say, "It's just suffering. It doesn't help."

Sometimes that's true—especially in chronic pain, where the signal has become distorted. But even distorted signals contain information. If you silence pain without understanding why it's there, you may gain short-term relief at the cost of long-term confusion.

This is the uncomfortable clinical truth: **pain is often a protective strategy.** But not necessarily an intelligent one. Not one we want forever. But a strategy, nonetheless.

If you numb it completely—whether with medication, repeated aggressive needling, constant adjustments, or any modality used like a hammer—you can remove the very feedback the body is using to limit further injury.

I've seen this play out in small and large ways:

- A patient with knee pain gets repeated injections, feels great, returns to aggressive sport, and two months later, the joint is worse. The pain wasn't the enemy—it was a speed limit being overridden.
- A patient with a back injury takes enough medication to work twelve-hour days through a flare. They "function," but their movement quality collapses. Months later, the whole region is locked, and the pain is now everywhere.
- A patient becomes dependent on weekly treatment not because it's the right interval for tissue change, but because it's the only time they feel safe.

This isn't an argument against symptom relief. People need

relief. Pain relief can restore sleep, reduce fear, and make movement possible again. That can be profoundly therapeutic.

The point is more subtle: **relief should not erase inquiry.**

A good treatment makes the patient feel better *and* makes the pattern clearer over time. It helps you both learn: What improves it? What worsens it? What kind of movement helps? What kind of rest helps? What kind of pressure, temperature, or activity changes the quality?

In other words, you're not just trying to get the pain score down. You're trying to increase information density.

And sometimes the most useful thing is not a dramatic reduction in pain, but a shift in its quality—sharp to dull, fixed to moving, cold to warm, deep to superficial, constant to intermittent. Those are not poetic descriptions. They are functional changes that tell you whether circulation is returning, whether guarding is easing, whether inflammation is changing phase, and whether the nervous system is lowering its threat response.

Suppressing pain without changing the underlying obstruction is like covering the dashboard lights with tape. The car may still run, but you've lost the warnings that help you drive wisely.

QI, BLOOD, AND FLUIDS: THREE WAYS OBSTRUCTION SHOWS UP

If pain is a failure of movement, what exactly is failing to move?

In classical Chinese medicine, we often speak of Qi, Blood, and fluids not as mystical substances, but as categories of function.

- **Qi** is coordination, signaling, warmth, tone, the capacity to initiate and regulate movement.
- **Blood** is nourishment, tissue perfusion, recovery, anchoring, the ability to soften and sustain.
- **Fluids** are lubrication, swelling dynamics, immune transport and the medium through which inflammation and resolution occur.

When any of these are impaired—or when their movement is constrained—pain emerges.

Qi stagnation: the grip, the knot, the constraint

Qi stagnation pain often feels tight, distending and changeable. It can move. It can be related to stress, frustration, pent-up emotion, or simply the nervous system stuck in a holding pattern. The person may sigh a lot, hold their breath without realizing it, clench their jaw, elevate their shoulders or brace their abdomen.

This is not "psychosomatic" in the dismissive sense. It's physiology. Autonomic tone alters blood flow, muscle tone, digestion, and inflammation. A person under chronic stress literally has less internal permission to release.

Qi stagnation pain often responds to:

- gentle movement and breath that restore rhythm
- warmth
- treatments that downshift vigilance (not just local needling, but regulating the whole pattern)
- strategies that reduce "all-or-nothing" activity cycles

But here's a trap: if you treat only Qi stagnation, you may temporarily loosen the grip while missing the underlying weakness that caused the body to grip in the first place. Sometimes the person is bracing because they don't trust their structure, their sleep is poor, their blood is insufficient, or their recovery capacity is low.

The stagnation can be protective.

Blood stasis: the fixed, stabbing, localized pain

Blood stasis pain is often more fixed, sharper, worse at night, and associated with a sensation of something being *stuck* in a particular place. There may be a history of trauma, surgery, repeated strain, or long-standing inflammation that has led to fibrosis and poor perfusion.

In the musculoskeletal world, "blood stasis" correlates with things like:

- persistent trigger points with ischemic tenderness
- old injuries that never fully regained elasticity
- adhesions and scar-related restrictions
- joints that feel thick, heavy, or locked

Blood stasis is not "bad blood." It's impaired microcirculation and tissue remodeling. And it's one reason chronic pain can persist long after the original injury: the tissues are not receiving what they need, and waste products are not clearing well.

Treating blood stasis can be powerful, but it also demands respect. If you move blood aggressively in a person who is depleted, you can create rebound pain, fatigue, bruising, and flare. The goal is not to "break it up" like a demolition crew. The goal is to restore intelligent perfusion.

Sometimes that means going slower than the patient wants.

Fluid obstruction: swelling, heaviness, damp congestion

Fluids are often overlooked in discussions of pain unless there's obvious edema. But fluid dynamics matter in everything from sinus pressure to joint effusions to nerve irritation.

Fluid congestion pain often feels heavy, swollen, dull and sometimes numb. It may worsen with humidity, certain foods, or inactivity. In joints, it can look like recurring effusion. In the head, it can feel like pressure or fog.

In inflammatory conditions, fluid stagnation can also reflect immune dysregulation: the body floods an area with inflammatory mediators but fails to resolve and clear them efficiently.

This is where the Chinese medicine category of "dampness" becomes clinically useful—again, not as a mystical pathogen, but as a way of describing congestion and impaired transformation.

A person with fluid obstruction often needs:

- improved metabolic and digestive support (because fluid handling is systemic)
- movement that stimulates lymphatic and venous return without overloading tissues
- warmth and rhythm
- sometimes gentle diuresis, sometimes production—depending on the pattern

And just as with Qi and Blood, the temptation is to "dry it out" aggressively. But if the person's fluids are congested because their system is weak, drying can worsen dryness, irritability, constipation, and sleep, leading to more pain.

Pain patterns are rarely pure Qi, pure Blood, or pure fluids. Most chronic pain is a braid.

The clinical art is to identify which strand can be pulled *right now* to get the best outcome, and what the system can tolerate.

RESTORING FLOW WITHOUT CHASING SENSATION

One of the easiest mistakes in pain treatment—especially with acupuncture and bodywork—is to chase sensation.

The patient says, "It hurts here," and the practitioner says, "Great, let's needle exactly there until it feels dramatic." Or they search for the most tender point and treat it as if tenderness is the target.

Sometimes local treatment is exactly right. There are moments when you need to meet the obstruction directly. But if you make intensity your compass, you can end up reinforcing the nervous system's fixation on the painful area.

I often tell patients: **We're not trying to win a fight against your pain. We're trying to change the environment that keeps pain necessary.**

That difference changes everything:

- You don't measure success by how intense the treatment felt.
- You don't measure success by whether the pain disappears on the table.
- You measure success by whether the person moves better afterward, sleeps better, recovers faster, and has fewer flares over time.

Restoring flow often means working *around* the pain—above and below, proximally and distally, systemically and locally—so the body can accept change without threat.

This is especially true in chronic pain with sensitization. If the nervous system has learned that a region is dangerous, aggressively manipulating it can confirm that belief. The person may feel temporarily "opened," then flare for three days. They come back saying, "It worked, but it made me worse." Then they ask for the same thing again because they're desperate. That is not a stable therapeutic loop.

A more mature strategy is to build capacity first:

- improve sleep
- reduce baseline inflammation
- regulate digestion and fluid handling
- restore a gentle range of motion
- reduce guarding through breath and tone work
- then gradually increase load and specificity

In acupuncture terms, this might mean choosing points that regulate the whole channel network rather than attacking the most painful spot. It might mean treating the constitutional pattern alongside the local region. It might mean fewer needles, less stimulation and more consistency.

In manual therapy, it might mean treating the ribcage and diaphragm for a neck problem, or the hip and foot for a knee problem—because movement is a chain, not a dot.

This can feel unsatisfying to people who want a quick fix. But in chronic pain, quick fixes often teach the nervous system to rely on external rescue rather than internal regulation.

And that brings us to an even more delicate point: pain is not only a tissue problem. It's a learning problem.

CHRONIC PAIN REQUIRES PATIENCE–BUT NOT PASSIVITY

"Be patient" is one of the least helpful things you can say to someone in pain.

It can sound like dismissal. It can sound like surrender. It can sound like, "Get used to it."

That's not what I mean.

I mean that chronic pain changes slowly because it is maintained by multiple interacting systems: local tissue condition, immune signaling, autonomic tone, fear circuits, sleep architecture, strength and coordination, habit loops and social context.

If you rush, you tend to treat only one layer—the loudest one—and the other layers stay intact. Then the pain returns, and everyone feels betrayed.

The alternative is not resignation. It's strategy.

Strategy looks like staging

Chronic pain care often happens in stages:

1. **Stabilize the flare cycle.**
2. Reduce frequency and intensity of spikes. Improve sleep. Help the patient feel less trapped.
3. **Restore basic movement without threat.**
4. Gentle range of motion, walking, breath-based regulation, and low-load strength. Not heroic rehab. Just rebuilding trust.
5. **Address deeper drivers.**
6. This might include hormonal patterns, inflammatory

foods, work ergonomics, unresolved injury mechanics, scar restrictions, emotional stress, or systemic deficiency.

7. **Build capacity and resilience.**
8. Return to meaningful activity gradually. Increase load tolerance. Teach pacing. Reduce fear of movement.
9. **Transition out of dependency.**
10. Treatment becomes less frequent, more self-directed. The patient owns the process.

Not every case follows this order neatly, but some version of staging is almost always required. Without staging, both the patient and the practitioner can end up in a frustrating cycle: treat a flare, flare returns, treat a flare, flare returns.

Strategy looks like choosing the right wins

In chronic pain, the best early wins are often not dramatic pain reductions. They are *functional* wins:

- "I slept through the night."
- "I walked for twenty minutes without anxiety about pain the next day."
- "My jaw is less clenched."
- "My period came with less back pain."
- "The pain moved instead of staying stuck."
- "When it flared, I knew what to do."

Those are the wins that create momentum. They teach the nervous system that change is possible and not dangerous.

And they protect the patient from the psychological collapse that chronic pain so often induces: the feeling that nothing helps, that the body is unreliable, that life is shrinking.

The goal is not to convince someone to tolerate pain. The goal is to expand their world again.

THE CLINICAL PARADOX: WE TREAT PAIN BEST WHEN WE STOP MAKING IT THE ONLY GOAL

It's reasonable for you to want pain gone. I want it gone, too. But when pain becomes the sole measure of success, it distorts decision-making.

Patients will overdo what helped once. Practitioners will over-apply what they're good at. Everyone will chase the most immediate reduction, even if it leads to a rebound.

In classical practice, we're trained—implicitly and explicitly—to treat *pattern*, not symptom. That can sound abstract. In pain care, it becomes very concrete.

A few examples from the clinic:

Example: The shoulder that "needs" deep work every week

A man in his forties with shoulder pain comes in after months of aggressive sports massage. He says deep pressure helps, but only for two days. Then the pain returns, and he books again.

On exam, his shoulder is guarded, his neck is rigid, and his breathing is shallow. He can't fully exhale. His sleep is light. He drinks coffee to push through fatigue. The shoulder is not the primary issue; it's the site where systemic tension expresses.

If I chase the shoulder with intensity, I might become his temporary relief provider. But if I treat the pattern—downregulate the system, improve sleep, restore breathing mechanics, reduce guarding—his shoulder no longer needs to scream for attention.

He may still need local work, but now it lands differently. It holds. He recovers.

This is not ideology. It's what happens when you stop rewarding the nervous system for escalating.

Example: The pelvic pain that worsens with "stronger treatment"

A woman with chronic pelvic pain has tried multiple modalities. She says acupuncture sometimes helps, but sometimes flares her badly. She's afraid of treatment now, but she's also desperate.

In cases like this, the pain system is often sensitized. The pelvis is a region where threat detection is already high because it relates to safety, sexuality, elimination and reproduction. Aggressive stimulation can amplify vigilance.

A treatment strategy that restores flow without chasing sensation might start far away: regulating sleep, digestion, and autonomic tone; using distal points; gentle abdominal work that prioritizes safety; slow exposure to movement; collaboration with pelvic floor therapy.

Over time, pain decreases—not because we "broke up stagnation," but because the system stopped interpreting normal sensation as danger.

Example: The back pain that improves when the patient stops being heroic

A person with chronic low back pain cycles between overactivity and collapse. On good days, they do everything. On bad days, they do nothing. The nervous system never finds a stable baseline.

This is where Chinese medicine's emphasis on rhythm becomes clinically relevant. We can support them with treatment, but the turning point often comes when they learn pacing: consistent, moderate movement; regular meals; regular sleep; fewer extremes.

Pain improves because movement becomes trustworthy again.

In each example, pain reduction is the result, but not the only target. The target is regulation.

THE ROLE OF PAIN IN TEACHING THE BODY—AND THE PERSON

Pain is not only something the body experiences. It's something the person interprets.

Two people can have similar tissue findings and completely different pain lives. One is frightened and constricted; the other is annoyed but mobile. One spirals into catastrophic thinking; the other adapts. One becomes dependent on external reassurance; the other learns to rely on internal cues.

This is not a character flaw. It's a learned relationship shaped by past experiences, trauma history, cultural messaging, medical encounters, and the nervous system's baseline tone.

So when we treat pain, we are also treating meaning.

That's why the clinical conversation matters as much as the needles or herbs.

A few principles I try to teach—quietly, repeatedly—because they build resilience:

1) Pain is a signal, not a verdict

A flare does not mean you are broken. It means the system exceeded its current capacity or encountered a trigger it hasn't learned to handle. If you treat every flare as evidence of permanent damage, fear becomes fuel.

If you treat flares as data—annoying data, sometimes miserable data—you can respond intelligently.

2) The goal is not to eliminate all sensation

Some patients try to reach a state where they feel nothing unusual in their body. That's not realistic. Healthy bodies have sensations. Aging bodies have sensations. Athletic bodies have sensations.

The goal is to reduce suffering and restore function, not to achieve numbness.

3) Capacity builds through tolerable exposure, not force

If you force through pain, you may win the moment and lose the month. If you avoid all discomfort, you may shrink your world until the nervous system becomes fragile.

The middle path—tolerable exposure—is where healing happens. This is as true for tendons and joints as it is for fear circuits.

4) Relief should increase autonomy, not dependency

This one is tender, because people in pain often feel powerless. The desire for rescue is human.

But the best clinical outcome is not a patient who needs you forever. It's a patient who uses you wisely when needed and can otherwise steer their own recovery.

When treatment creates dependency—weekly forever, panic if they miss, fear of self-management—it may reduce pain temporarily, but it increases vulnerability.

A mature practice aims for the opposite: decreasing frequency over time, increasing self-efficacy, and increasing understanding. The endgame is a patient who happily lives their life without the need for external regulation. In practice, this looks like annual or quarterly visits to make sure their system is doing well.

That doesn't mean abandoning patients. It means teaching them how to maintain and grow their gains.

WHAT "RESTORING FLOW" LOOKS LIKE IN REAL LIFE

"Restore flow" can sound vague until you translate it into lived behaviors and measurable changes.

In pain care, restoring flow tends to show up as:

- **Better circulation**: warmth returns to cold areas; tissues feel less ropey; pain shifts from fixed to mobile.
- **Better variability**: the body can tense and relax again; the person can move without holding breath.
- **Better recovery**: post-activity soreness resolves faster; flares shorten.
- **Better sleep**: fewer wake-ups; less early morning stiffness; better dreams.
- **Better digestion**: less bloating; more regular bowel movements; steadier appetite and energy.
- **Better mood and cognition**: less irritability, less dread, more clarity.

None of these are mystical. They're signs that the organism is regaining regulatory range.

In Chinese medicine language, you might say Qi is moving, Blood is nourishing, and fluids are transforming. But you can also say: the nervous system is less threatened, the tissues are perfused, inflammation resolves more efficiently, and the person is breathing.

A note on "moving stagnation" in chronic pain

There is a common temptation—especially among practitioners early in their career—to treat chronic pain as a problem that needs aggressive movement: strong stimulation, strong herbs, strong techniques.

Sometimes that's exactly what's needed. But chronic pain patients often have less reserve than they appear to have. Their system has been spending fuel on vigilance for a long time. When you push too hard, you can create a flare that reinforces the idea that change is dangerous.

The paradox is that the most effective "moving" treatments are often the ones that the body can integrate.

That requires restraint. It requires listening. It requires allowing the patient to improve at a pace that feels steady rather than dramatic.

ACUTE VERSUS CHRONIC: DIFFERENT CONVERSATIONS, DIFFERENT CONTRACTS

One of the most important parts of pain care is setting the right expectations—without making promises you can't keep.

With acute pain, the conversation is often:

- "We need to calm this down."
- "We need to protect the area while it heals."
- "We're watching for red flags."
- "You should improve week by week."

With chronic pain, the conversation shifts:

- "We're going to change the trend."
- "We're going to reduce flares and increase capacity."
- "We're going to build a plan that you can live with."
- "This can improve, but we don't know how much. Yet."

This is not pessimism. It's respect for the complexity of chronic pain.

Patients often feel relief when you tell the truth calmly. Many have been bounced between extremes: either "nothing is wrong" or "you're damaged forever." A more accurate message is usually: something is happening, it makes sense, and we can work with it.

TEACHING RESILIENCE INSTEAD OF DEPENDENCY

If there is one ethical thread I want to pull through pain medicine, it's this: **the goal is not to keep patients in care. The goal is to return them to their life.**

That doesn't mean the relationship ends. Some people with complex conditions will always benefit from periodic support. But the direction should be toward agency.

Resilience is not grit. It's not "toughen up." It's not ignoring pain.

Resilience is:

- knowing how to respond to early signals
- having tools that work predictably
- trusting your ability to recover
- having a plan for flares that doesn't involve panic
- maintaining meaningful activity without self-punishment

In practice, this might look like:

- Teaching a patient to distinguish "good soreness" from warning pain.
- Helping them find the minimum effective dose of treatment—then spacing visits.
- Giving them one or two exercises they can actually do consistently, rather than a fantasy program.
- Teaching breath patterns that downshift guarding.
- Helping them track patterns without becoming obsessive.
- Naming the flare cycle so they stop interpreting it as personal failure.

It's also about boundaries—on both sides.

Patients sometimes want the practitioner to be the manager of their body. Practitioners sometimes enjoy being needed. Neither leads to the best outcomes.

A healthier contract is collaborative: I help you see the map, we test interventions, you learn what works, and over time, you rely more on your own capacity than on my hands.

This is no less caring. It's deeper care.

CLOSING: PAIN AS OBSTRUCTION, PAIN AS INVITATION

Pain narrows the world. It makes people smaller. It pulls attention into a single region, a single fear, a single question: "How do I make this stop?"

A good clinician helps widen the frame. We work to minimize their suffering by broadening their horizons, whether or not we can lower their pain.

When we understand pain as obstruction and message, we stop treating it as a moral problem ("you're weak"), a mechanical problem alone ("you're broken"), or a nuisance to suppress at all costs ("just make it quiet"). We treat it as a living signal arising from a system that is trying—often clumsily—to protect itself.

Sometimes the message is simple: stop, heal, don't ignore this. Sometimes the message is more complex: you've been bracing for years, your sleep is thin, your digestion is strained, your tissues are undernourished, your nervous system is on watch, and the body is asking for a new way to move through life.

Restoring flow is not glamorous. It is often slow, repetitive, and unremarkable from the outside. But it is how chronic pain actually changes: not by conquering sensation, but by rebuilding regulation.

And when that happens, something quietly profound occurs. The person doesn't just hurt less. They fear less. They move more. They trust their body again.

That trust—more than any single technique—is the beginning of real healing.

12

Pain as Obstruction and Message

Pain makes people honest.

Not morally—clinically. Pain has a way of stripping away the stories we tell ourselves about what we can tolerate, what we should ignore, what we can push through. It forces the nervous system to speak up. It reorganizes priorities. It changes posture, breath, sleep, mood, appetite, relationship. And it brings people into the clinic who have been "fine" for years—until they weren't.

The problem is that pain also makes people reactive. Patients want it gone yesterday. Practitioners want to fix it quickly, partly out of compassion and partly because no one likes to sit with a suffering person and say, "This will take time." Entire medical systems are designed around rapid suppression because it's measurable and marketable: pain score down, job done.

But Chinese medicine—at least in its older, clinically serious forms—doesn't treat pain as an enemy to be silenced. It treats pain as information about movement.

That doesn't mean we romanticize it. Pain is not "a teacher" in the motivational-poster sense. It's often brutal, limiting, and demoralizing. Some pain is dangerous and demands urgent care. Some pain is senseless—injury, degeneration, based on damage. And some pain persists long after tissues have technically "healed," because the nervous system has changed its rules.

Still, pain is rarely random. It has shape. It has timing. It has a relationship with rest, with weather, with stress, with digestion, with sleep, with menstrual cycles, with breathing, with fear. It has patterns.

If you can read those patterns, pain becomes less mysterious—and less tyrannical. Not because you've learned a trick, but because you've learned what it's pointing to.

This chapter is about that: pain as a failure of movement, pain as obstruction, pain as message. And what it means to treat pain without becoming trapped by it.

PAIN IS OFTEN A FAILURE OF MOVEMENT —NOT A THING IN ITSELF

A common modern framing is: pain equals tissue damage. If something hurts, something must be broken.

That's sometimes true. A fracture hurts for a reason. Appendicitis hurts for a reason. An infection hurts for a reason. There are pains you do not negotiate with.

But a surprising amount of pain—especially musculoskeletal pain, headache patterns, pelvic pain, many types of neuropathic pain—doesn't correlate cleanly with tissue damage. People have terrible MRIs and no pain, and "normal" imaging with debilitating pain. Even when damage exists, it often doesn't explain the full intensity or persistence.

Classical Chinese medicine starts from a different assumption: pain is frequently what happens when normal movement is interrupted.

Movement here doesn't just mean joint range of motion. It means the ability of a region, a tissue, or a system to do its job without strain: to circulate, to warm and cool appropriately, to repair, to adapt, to transition from tension to relaxation and back again.

When movement is reduced, the body doesn't merely lose function. It becomes louder. The nervous system increases surveillance. Local tissues become sensitive. Muscles brace. Breathing changes. The area becomes precious and guarded. And pain becomes a kind of protective alarm—sometimes appropriate, sometimes excessive.

In older language, you'll hear, "Where there is obstruction, there is pain. Where there is free flow, there is no pain." That line gets repeated so often it can feel like a slogan. The deeper value is this: it invites you to look for *what is not moving*.

- Is the joint itself mechanically restricted?
- Is the fascia stiff, densified, protective?
- Is blood flow cold, ischemic, slow to recover?
- Is fluid movement swelling, edema, inflammatory congestion?
- Is nerve function inflamed, irritated, hypersensitive?
- Is the person trapped in bracing, unable to exhale, unable to soften?

Pain often lives at the boundary between what the body is asking for and what the person is forcing.

One of the most useful clinical questions I know is deceptively simple: **What movement is being prevented—locally or systemically?**

Sometimes it's literal. A frozen shoulder hurts because the capsule has tightened and the brain has learned to protect it. A neck that can't rotate hurts because the surrounding tissues have become vigilant. A pelvic floor that can't release hurts because the body has decided that release is unsafe.

Sometimes it's less literal. Someone with migraines that come every Sunday night might not have "a head problem" at all. They might have a week-long buildup of sympathetic drive and poor eating, followed by a sudden drop in adrenaline and a rebound vascular and inflammatory response. The pain is the endpoint of a weekly rhythm that's become pathological.

In that sense, pain is not a thing you treat. It's a relationship you change.

ACUTE PAIN AND CHRONIC PAIN ARE NOT THE SAME PROBLEM

If you treat all pain the same way, you'll either under-treat danger or over-treat adaptation.

In the clinic, I separate pain into two broad categories—not because life is that tidy, but because decision-making improves when you respect the difference:

Acute pain: the alarm that matches the moment

Acute pain is often tied to a recent event: injury, infection, surgical trauma, sudden inflammation, a clear flare of arthritis, a kidney stone, a disc protrusion, an acute nerve irritation.

The key features are:

- It has a relatively clear onset.
- It changes rapidly.
- It often responds to appropriate rest and protection.
- It often comes with signs of active tissue threat: heat, swelling, sharpness, redness, fever, night pain that's new and escalating.

In Chinese medicine terms, acute pain often involves more obvious excess: sudden obstruction, heat, swelling, spasm. The body is mobilizing resources, and the system is loud.

The goal here is not heroic. It is intelligent containment: calm the acute threat, keep the person safe, prevent maladaptive guarding from becoming the new normal, and support recovery. You don't want to "power through" acute pain, but you also don't want to freeze a person into immobility for weeks unless that's truly necessary.

This is where good triage matters. Some acute pain needs imaging, labs, emergency care. Chinese medicine is not a substitute for that. A clinician who treats severe new pain as "just stagnation" is not practicing medicine—they're practicing denial.

Chronic pain: the alarm that has rewritten the rules

Chronic pain is different. It may begin acutely, but then it persists beyond the expected tissue healing time. Or it may creep in gradually, woven into years of posture, stress, sleep debt, inflammation, and micro-injuries.

Chronic pain tends to have:

- A history of flare and remission.
- Triggers that include stress, weather, fatigue, certain foods, poor sleep.
- A strong relationship to mood, attention, and fear (not because it's "in the mind," but because the nervous system is involved).
- A pattern of compensation: one area hurts, then another takes over and starts hurting too.

In Chinese medicine terms, chronic pain is rarely a single excess. It's often a layered pattern: obstruction plus deficiency, stagnation plus weakness, local congestion plus systemic inability to resolve it. The loudness of pain can coexist with low reserves.

This is where simplistic approaches backfire—especially approaches that chase the loudest symptom. We've already talked earlier in the book about how over-clearing or over-warming can create second- and third-order problems. Chronic pain is one of the places that lesson matters most.

In chronic pain, the goal is not simply to "turn pain off." The goal is to change the conditions that keep pain necessary.

That takes time. And it requires a different kind of therapeutic relationship—one that treats the patient as an adaptive organism, not a broken machine.

WHEN YOU SUPPRESS PAIN TOO SUCCESSFULLY, YOU LOSE THE MAP

Pain has a reputation for being useless. People say, "It's just suffering. It doesn't help."

Sometimes that's true—especially in chronic pain, where the signal has become distorted. But even distorted signals contain information. If you silence pain without understanding why it's there, you may gain short-term relief at the cost of long-term confusion.

This is the uncomfortable clinical truth: **pain is often a protective strategy.** But not necessarily an intelligent one. Not one we want forever. But a strategy nonetheless.

If you numb it completely—whether with medication, repeated aggressive needling, constant adjustments, or any modality used like a hammer—you can remove the very feedback the body is using to limit further injury.

I've seen this play out in small and large ways:

- A patient with knee pain gets repeated injections, feels great, returns to aggressive sport, and two months later, the joint is worse. The pain wasn't the enemy—it was a speed limit being overridden.
- A patient with a back injury takes enough medication to work twelve-hour days through a flare. They "function," but their movement quality collapses. Months later, the whole region is locked, and the pain is now everywhere.
- A patient becomes dependent on weekly treatment not because it's the right interval for tissue change, but because it's the only time they feel safe.

This isn't an argument against symptom relief. People need relief. Pain relief can restore sleep, reduce fear, and make movement possible again. That can be profoundly therapeutic.

The point is more subtle: **relief should not erase inquiry.**

A good treatment makes the patient feel better *and* makes the pattern clearer over time. It helps you both learn: What improves it?

What worsens it? What kind of movement helps? What kind of rest helps? What kind of pressure, temperature, or activity changes the quality?

In other words, you're not just trying to get the pain score down. You're trying to get information density up.

And sometimes the most useful thing is not a dramatic reduction in pain, but a shift in its quality—sharp to dull, fixed to moving, cold to warm, deep to superficial, constant to intermittent. Those are not poetic descriptions. They are functional changes that tell you whether circulation is returning, whether guarding is easing, whether inflammation is changing phase, whether the nervous system is lowering its threat response.

Suppressing pain without changing the underlying obstruction is like covering the dashboard lights with tape. The car may still run, but you've lost the warnings that help you drive wisely.

QI, BLOOD, AND FLUIDS: THREE WAYS OBSTRUCTION SHOWS UP

If pain is a failure of movement, what exactly is failing to move?

In classical Chinese medicine, we often speak of Qi, Blood, and fluids not as mystical substances, but as categories of function.

- **Qi** is coordination, signaling, warmth, tone, the capacity to initiate and regulate movement.
- **Blood** is nourishment, tissue perfusion, recovery, anchoring, the ability to soften and sustain.
- **Fluids** are lubrication, swelling dynamics, immune transport, the medium through which inflammation and resolution occur.

When any of these are impaired—or when their movement is constrained—pain emerges.

Qi stagnation: the grip, the knot, the constraint

Qi stagnation pain often feels tight, distending, changeable. It can move. It can be related to stress, frustration, pent-up emotion, or simply the nervous system stuck in a holding pattern. The person may sigh a lot, hold their breath without realizing it, clench their jaw, elevate their shoulders, brace their abdomen.

This is not "psychosomatic" in the dismissive sense. It's physiology. Autonomic tone alters blood flow, muscle tone, digestion, and inflammation. A person under chronic stress literally has less internal permission to release.

Qi stagnation pain often responds to:

- gentle movement and breath that restore rhythm
- warmth
- treatments that downshift vigilance (not just local needling, but regulating the whole pattern)
- strategies that reduce "all-or-nothing" activity cycles

But here's a trap: if you treat only Qi stagnation, you may temporarily loosen the grip while missing the underlying weakness that caused the body to grip in the first place. Sometimes the person is bracing because they don't trust their structure, their sleep is poor, their blood is insufficient, or their recovery capacity is low.

The stagnation can be protective.

Blood stasis: the fixed, stabbing, localized pain

Blood stasis pain is often more fixed, sharper, worse at night, and associated with a sense that something is *stuck* in a particular place. There may be a history of trauma, surgery, repeated strain, or long-standing inflammation that has led to fibrosis and poor perfusion.

In the musculoskeletal world, "blood stasis" correlates with things like:

- persistent trigger points with ischemic tenderness

- old injuries that never fully regained elasticity
- adhesions and scar-related restrictions
- joints that feel thick, heavy, or locked

Blood stasis is not "bad blood." It's impaired microcirculation and tissue remodeling. And it's one reason chronic pain can persist long after the original injury: the tissues are not receiving what they need, and waste products are not clearing well.

Treating blood stasis can be powerful, but it also demands respect. If you move blood aggressively in a person who is depleted, you can create rebound pain, fatigue, bruising, and flare. The goal is not to "break it up" like a demolition crew. The goal is to restore intelligent perfusion.

Sometimes that means going slower than the patient wants.

Fluid obstruction: swelling, heaviness, damp congestion

Fluids are often overlooked in pain discussions unless there's obvious edema. But fluid dynamics matter in everything from sinus pressure to joint effusions to nerve irritation.

Fluid congestion pain often feels heavy, swollen, dull, sometimes numb. It may worsen with humidity, certain foods, or inactivity. In joints, it can look like recurring effusion. In the head, it can feel like pressure or fog.

In inflammatory conditions, fluid stagnation can also reflect immune dysregulation: the body floods an area with inflammatory mediators but fails to resolve and clear them efficiently.

This is where the Chinese medicine category of "dampness" becomes clinically useful—again, not as a mystical pathogen, but as a way of describing congestion and impaired transformation.

A person with fluid obstruction often needs:

- improved metabolic and digestive support (because fluid handling is systemic)

- movement that stimulates lymphatic and venous return without overloading tissues
- warmth and rhythm
- sometimes gentle diuresis, sometimes production—depending on the pattern

And just as with Qi and Blood, the temptation is to "dry it out" aggressively. But if the person's fluids are congested because their system is weak, drying can worsen dryness, irritability, constipation, and sleep—leading to more pain.

Pain patterns are rarely pure Qi, pure Blood, or pure fluids. Most chronic pain is a braid.

The clinical art is to identify which strand can be pulled *right now* to get the best outcome, and what the system can tolerate.

RESTORING FLOW WITHOUT CHASING SENSATION

One of the easiest mistakes in pain treatment—especially with acupuncture and bodywork—is to chase sensation.

The patient says, "It hurts here," and the practitioner says, "Great, let's needle exactly there until it feels dramatic." Or they search for the most tender point and treat it as if tenderness is the target.

Sometimes local treatment is exactly right. There are moments when you need to meet the obstruction directly. But if you make intensity your compass, you can end up reinforcing the nervous system's fixation on the painful area.

I often tell patients: **We're not trying to win a fight against your pain. We're trying to change the environment that keeps pain necessary.**

That difference changes everything:

- You don't measure success by how intense the treatment felt.

- You don't measure success by whether the pain disappears on the table.
- You measure success by whether the person moves better afterward, sleeps better, recovers faster, and has fewer flares over time.

Restoring flow often means working *around* the pain—above and below, proximally and distally, systemically and locally—so the body can accept change without threat.

This is especially true in chronic pain with sensitization. If the nervous system has learned that a region is dangerous, aggressively manipulating it can confirm that belief. The person may feel temporarily "opened," then flare for three days. They come back saying, "It worked, but it made me worse." Then they ask for the same thing again because they're desperate. That is not a stable therapeutic loop.

A more mature strategy is to build capacity first:

- improve sleep
- reduce baseline inflammation
- regulate digestion and fluid handling
- restore a gentle range of motion
- reduce guarding through breath and tone work
- then gradually increase load and specificity

In acupuncture terms, this might mean choosing points that regulate the whole channel network rather than attacking the most painful spot. It might mean treating the constitutional pattern alongside the local region. It might mean fewer needles, less stimulation, more consistency.

In manual therapy, it might mean treating the ribcage and diaphragm for a neck problem, or the hip and foot for a knee problem—because movement is a chain, not a dot.

This can feel unsatisfying to people who want a quick fix. But in chronic pain, quick fixes often teach the nervous system to rely on external rescue rather than internal regulation.

And that brings us to an even more delicate point: pain is not only a tissue problem. It's a learning problem.

CHRONIC PAIN REQUIRES PATIENCE—BUT NOT PASSIVITY

"Be patient" is one of the least helpful things you can say to someone in pain.

It can sound like dismissal. It can sound like surrender. It can sound like, "Get used to it."

That's not what I mean.

I mean that chronic pain changes slowly because it is maintained by multiple interacting systems: local tissue condition, immune signaling, autonomic tone, fear circuits, sleep architecture, strength and coordination, habit loops, social context.

If you rush, you tend to treat only one layer—the loudest one—and the other layers stay intact. Then the pain returns, and everyone feels betrayed.

The alternative is not resignation. It's strategy.

Strategy looks like staging

Chronic pain care often happens in stages:

1. **Stabilize the flare cycle.**
2. Reduce frequency and intensity of spikes. Improve sleep. Help the patient feel less trapped.
3. **Restore basic movement without threat.**
4. Gentle range of motion, walking, breath-based regulation, low-load strength. Not heroic rehab. Just rebuilding trust.
5. **Address deeper drivers.**
6. This might include hormonal patterns, inflammatory foods, work ergonomics, unresolved injury mechanics, scar restrictions, emotional stress, or systemic deficiency.
7. **Build capacity and resilience.**

8. Return to meaningful activity gradually. Increase load tolerance. Teach pacing. Reduce fear of movement.
9. **Transition out of dependency.**
10. Treatment becomes less frequent, more self-directed. The patient owns the process.

Not every case follows this order neatly, but some version of staging is almost always required. Without staging, both patient and practitioner can end up in a frustrating cycle: treat flare, flare returns, treat flare, flare returns.

Strategy looks like choosing the right wins

In chronic pain, the best early wins are often not dramatic pain reductions. They are *functional* wins:

- "I slept through the night."
- "I walked for twenty minutes without anxiety about pain the next day."
- "My jaw is less clenched."
- "My period came with less back pain."
- "The pain moved instead of staying stuck."
- "When it flared, I knew what to do."

Those are the wins that create momentum. They teach the nervous system that change is possible and not dangerous.

And they protect the patient from the psychological collapse that chronic pain so often induces: the feeling that nothing helps, that the body is unreliable, that life is shrinking.

The goal is not to convince someone to tolerate pain. The goal is to expand their world again.

THE CLINICAL PARADOX: WE TREAT PAIN BEST WHEN WE STOP MAKING IT THE ONLY GOAL

It's reasonable for you to want pain gone. I want it gone, too. But when pain becomes the sole measure of success, it distorts decision-making.

Patients will overdo what helped once. Practitioners will over-apply what they're good at. Everyone will chase the most immediate reduction, even if it leads to a rebound.

In classical practice, we're trained—implicitly and explicitly—to treat *pattern*, not symptom. That can sound abstract. In pain care, it becomes very concrete.

A few examples from the clinic:

Example: The shoulder that "needs" deep work every week

A man in his forties with shoulder pain comes in after months of aggressive sports massage. He says deep pressure helps, but only for two days. Then the pain returns, and he books again.

On exam, his shoulder is guarded, his neck is rigid, his breathing is shallow. He can't fully exhale. His sleep is light. He drinks coffee to push through fatigue. The shoulder is not the primary issue; it's the site where systemic tension expresses.

If I chase the shoulder with intensity, I might become his temporary relief provider. But if I treat the pattern—downregulate the system, improve sleep, restore breathing mechanics, reduce guarding—his shoulder stops needing to scream for attention.

He may still need local work, but now it lands differently. It holds. He recovers.

This is not ideology. It's what happens when you stop rewarding the nervous system for escalating.

Example: The pelvic pain that worsens with "stronger treatment"

A woman with chronic pelvic pain has tried multiple modalities. She says acupuncture sometimes helps but sometimes flares her badly. She's afraid of treatment now, but she's also desperate.

In cases like this, the pain system is often sensitized. The pelvis is a region where threat detection is already high because it relates to safety, sexuality, elimination, reproduction. Aggressive stimulation can amplify vigilance.

A treatment strategy that restores flow without chasing sensation might start far away: regulating sleep, digestion, and autonomic tone; using distal points; gentle abdominal work that prioritizes safety; slow exposure to movement; collaboration with pelvic floor therapy.

Over time, pain decreases—not because we "broke up stagnation," but because the system stopped interpreting normal sensation as danger.

Example: The back pain that improves when the patient stops being heroic

A person with chronic low back pain cycles between overactivity and collapse. On good days they do everything. On bad days they do nothing. The nervous system never finds a stable baseline.

This is where Chinese medicine's emphasis on rhythm becomes clinically relevant. We can support them with treatment, but the turning point often comes when they learn pacing: consistent, moderate movement; regular meals; regular sleep; fewer extremes.

Pain improves because movement becomes trustworthy again.

In each example, pain reduction is the result, but not the only target. The target is regulation.

THE ROLE OF PAIN IN TEACHING THE BODY—AND THE PERSON

Pain is not only something the body experiences. It's something the person interprets.

Two people can have similar tissue findings and completely different pain lives. One is frightened and constricted; the other is annoyed but mobile. One spirals into catastrophic thinking; the other adapts. One becomes dependent on external reassurance; the other learns internal cues.

This is not a character flaw. It's a learned relationship shaped by past experiences, trauma history, cultural messaging, medical encounters, and the nervous system's baseline tone.

So when we treat pain, we are also treating meaning.

That's why the clinical conversation matters as much as the needles or herbs.

A few principles I try to teach—quietly, repeatedly—because they build resilience:

1) Pain is a signal, not a verdict

A flare does not mean you are broken. It means the system exceeded its current capacity or encountered a trigger it hasn't learned to handle. If you treat every flare as evidence of permanent damage, fear becomes fuel.

If you treat flares as data—annoying data, sometimes miserable data—you can respond intelligently.

2) The goal is not to eliminate all sensation

Some patients try to reach a state where they feel nothing unusual in their body. That's not realistic. Healthy bodies have sensations. Aging bodies have sensations. Athletic bodies have sensations.

The goal is to reduce suffering and restore function, not to achieve numbness.

3) Capacity builds through tolerable exposure, not force

If you force through pain, you may win the moment and lose the month. If you avoid all discomfort, you may shrink your world until the nervous system becomes fragile.

The middle path—tolerable exposure—is where healing happens. This is as true for tendons and joints as it is for fear circuits.

4) Relief should increase autonomy, not dependency

This one is tender, because people in pain often feel powerless. The desire for rescue is human.

But the best clinical outcome is not a patient who needs you forever. It's a patient who uses you wisely when needed and can otherwise steer their own recovery.

When treatment creates dependency—weekly forever, panic if they miss, fear of self-management—it may reduce pain temporarily, but it increases vulnerability.

A mature practice aims for the opposite: decreasing frequency over time, increasing self-efficacy, increasing understanding. The endgame is a patient who happily lives their life without the need for external regulation. In practice, this looks like annual or quarterly visits to make sure their system is doing well.

That doesn't mean abandoning patients. It means teaching them how to maintain and grow their gains.

WHAT "RESTORING FLOW" LOOKS LIKE IN REAL LIFE

"Restore flow" can sound vague until you translate it into lived behaviors and measurable changes.

In pain care, restoring flow tends to show up as:

- **Better circulation**: warmth returns to cold areas; tissues feel less ropey; pain shifts from fixed to mobile.
- **Better variability**: the body can tense and relax again; the person can move without holding breath.
- **Better recovery**: post-activity soreness resolves faster; flares shorten.
- **Better sleep**: fewer wake-ups; less early morning stiffness; better dreams.
- **Better digestion**: less bloating; more regular bowel movements; steadier appetite and energy.
- **Better mood and cognition**: less irritability, less dread, more clarity.

None of these are mystical. They're signs that the organism is regaining regulatory range.

In Chinese medicine language, you might say Qi is moving, Blood is nourishing, fluids are transforming. But you can also say: the nervous system is less threatened, the tissues are perfused, inflammation resolves more efficiently, the person is breathing.

A note on "moving stagnation" in chronic pain

There is a common temptation—especially among practitioners early in their career—to treat chronic pain as a problem that needs aggressive movement: strong stimulation, strong herbs, strong techniques.

Sometimes that's exactly what's needed. But chronic pain patients often have less reserve than they appear to have. Their system has been spending fuel on vigilance for a long time. When you push too hard, you can create a flare that reinforces the idea that change is dangerous.

The paradox is that the most effective "moving" treatments are often the ones that the body can integrate.

That requires restraint. It requires listening. It requires letting the patient improve at a pace that doesn't feel dramatic but is stable.

ACUTE VERSUS CHRONIC: DIFFERENT CONVERSATIONS, DIFFERENT CONTRACTS

One of the most important parts of pain care is setting the right expectations—without making promises you can't keep.

With acute pain, the conversation is often:

- "We need to calm this down."
- "We need to protect the area while it heals."
- "We're watching for red flags."
- "You should improve week by week."

With chronic pain, the conversation shifts:

- "We're going to change the trend."
- "We're going to reduce flares and increase capacity."
- "We're going to build a plan that you can live with."
- "This can improve, but we don't know how much. Yet."

This is not pessimism. It's respect for the complexity of chronic pain.

Patients often feel relief when you tell the truth calmly. Many have been bounced between extremes: either "nothing is wrong" or "you're damaged forever." A more accurate message is usually: something is happening, it makes sense, and we can work with it.

TEACHING RESILIENCE INSTEAD OF DEPENDENCY

If there is one ethical thread I want to pull through pain medicine, it's this: **the goal is not to keep patients in care. The goal is to return them to their life.**

That doesn't mean the relationship ends. Some people with complex conditions will always benefit from periodic support. But the direction should be toward agency.

Resilience is not grit. It's not "toughen up." It's not ignoring pain.

Resilience is:

- knowing how to respond to early signals
- having tools that work predictably
- trusting your ability to recover
- having a plan for flares that doesn't involve panic
- maintaining meaningful activity without self-punishment

In practice, this might look like:

- Teaching a patient to distinguish "good soreness" from warning pain.
- Helping them find the minimum effective dose of treatment—then spacing visits.
- Giving them one or two exercises they can actually do consistently, rather than a fantasy program.
- Teaching breath patterns that downshift guarding.
- Helping them track patterns without becoming obsessive.
- Naming the flare cycle so they stop interpreting it as personal failure.

It's also about boundaries—on both sides.

Patients sometimes want the practitioner to be the manager of their body. Practitioners sometimes enjoy being needed. Neither leads to the best outcomes.

A healthier contract is collaborative: I help you see the map, we test interventions, you learn what works, and over time you rely more on your own capacity than on my hands.

This is no less caring. It's deeper care.

CLOSING: PAIN AS OBSTRUCTION, PAIN AS INVITATION

Pain narrows the world. It makes people smaller. It pulls attention into a single region, a single fear, a single question: "How do I make this stop?"

A good clinician helps widen the frame. We work to minimize their suffering by broadening their horizons, whether or not we can lower their pain.

When we understand pain as obstruction and message, we stop treating it as a moral problem ("you're weak"), a mechanical problem alone ("you're broken"), or a nuisance to suppress at all costs ("just make it quiet"). We treat it as a living signal arising from a system that is trying—often clumsily—to protect itself.

Sometimes the message is simple: stop, heal, don't ignore this. Sometimes the message is more complex: you've been bracing for years, your sleep is thin, your digestion is strained, your tissues are undernourished, your nervous system is on watch, and the body is asking for a new way to move through life.

Restoring flow is not glamorous. It is often slow, repetitive, and unremarkable from the outside. But it is how chronic pain actually changes: not by conquering sensation, but by rebuilding regulation.

And when that happens, something quietly profound occurs. The person doesn't just hurt less. They fear less. They move more. They trust their body again.

That trust—more than any single technique—is the beginning of real healing.

13

What This Medicine Knows

There is a question worth asking at the end of any book that has asked you to think differently: What do you actually take with you?

Not the terminology. Not the frameworks as frameworks. But the ideas underneath, the ones that change how you see a body, how you listen to a symptom, how you decide what matters in a clinical encounter or in your own health. The ones that, once you've absorbed them, make it difficult to go back to the simpler version.

This book has covered a lot of terrain. But it has really only been making five arguments. They have been present in every chapter, approached from different angles, and tested against different clinical problems. This final chapter isn't a summary. It's an attempt to say plainly what those five arguments are and why they matter beyond Chinese medicine.

THE BODY IS TRYING TO DO SOMETHING

The first argument is the most foundational and, in some ways, the most subversive.

When something goes wrong in the body (pain, fatigue, insomnia, inflammation that won't resolve), the natural instinct is to ask: What is malfunctioning? What is broken? Where is the defect?

Chinese medicine starts somewhere different. It asks: What is the body trying to accomplish, and what is preventing it from accomplishing it cleanly?

That shift sounds subtle, but its clinical consequences run deep. If you treat a symptom as a malfunction, your job is to suppress it. If you treat a symptom as the body's best available solution to a problem it cannot otherwise solve, your job becomes more complicated and more interesting. You have to ask what the symptom is solving. What would happen if you removed it without addressing the underlying pressure it's responding to?

You've seen this throughout the book. Chronic pain that guards an unstable joint. A fever coordinates the immune response. Insomnia that keeps a person from descending into feelings they haven't had room to process. Diarrhea that evacuates something the gut cannot tolerate. None of these is a failure in the usual sense. They are strategies, sometimes maladaptive, often expensive, always attempting coherence.

This doesn't mean we leave suffering in place out of philosophical respect for its logic. It means we treat more intelligently when we know what we're overriding. A treatment that silences the symptom without changing the underlying condition isn't a cure. It's a temporary management of something that will eventually find another form.

We watch this play out in the clinic constantly. A patient's reflux improves with medication, but their sleep worsens. Someone's anxiety quiets with sedation, but their digestion collapses. Another patient's inflammation is suppressed, but their fatigue deepens. The body didn't stop trying to solve its problem; it just found a different way to express it.

The body is consistent. It follows rules. It does not malfunction randomly. And when you stop looking for defects and start looking for logic, the case that seemed like a mystery often becomes legible.

CHRONIC ILLNESS IS A PATTERN, NOT A LOCATION

The second argument follows directly from the first, and it requires something of the clinician that our medical infrastructure doesn't always support: the willingness to hold the whole picture at once.

Think of the patient we've met in various forms throughout this book. Migraines, jaw clenching, reflux, waking at 3 a.m., and premenstrual irritability. In a symptom-based frame, that's five problems, five referrals, five partial explanations. But you already know what that looks like from the inside: one pattern with five addresses. The body is not failing in five places simultaneously. It is organized around a disruption that manifests in five places simultaneously.

This is the clinical gift of pattern recognition: it gives you a lever, not a checklist. When you see the pattern underneath the scatter, you stop asking which of these five things to treat first and start asking which intervention will shift the whole system at once. The answer is often simpler than you'd expect, and often located somewhere other than where the loudest symptom is.

The corollary matters just as much. Two patients with the same diagnosis do not necessarily share the same pattern. We talked about this with knee pain: the same complaint arising from digestion, emotion, constitution, or constraint. The diagnosis names the category; the pattern describes the living physiology: same label, different terrain, different treatment.

This can feel counterintuitive to a medical culture organized around the idea that the same disease should receive the same protocol. What Chinese medicine offers here is not relativism. It's precision at a different level. Not the precision of targeting a single mechanism, but the precision of identifying which functional disruption is generating this whole cluster in this particular person. That kind of precision requires more from the clinician, but it also produces more durable results, because it treats the organization rather than its outputs.

WHERE YOU INTERVENE ON THE TIMELINE CHANGES EVERYTHING

The third argument is the one modern medicine is slowly arriving at through its own routes, and it may be the one with the most practical urgency.

Function shifts before structure does. We've returned to this idea throughout the book because it keeps showing up in real cases. The body begins to behave differently (sleeping differently, digesting differently, regulating temperature differently, recovering differently) before any of those changes become visible on a scan or measurable in a lab value.

That functional territory is not a waiting room before the "real" illness arrives. It is a phase in which the system is still plastic, still negotiating, still capable of reorganization without major force. Working in that territory is not alternative medicine. It is early medicine.

The classical tradition built its entire diagnostic language around reading those early signals: pulse, tongue, the close attention to symptom quality, timing and context. It did so precisely because that is where change is still relatively inexpensive, where a nudge can redirect a trajectory that, left alone, will require a much larger intervention several years later.

This has implications for how we think about prevention, which is usually framed as the absence of behavior: don't smoke, don't drink, don't eat this. That is one kind of prevention. But there is another kind, more active, more clinical, more interesting: the early recognition that a system is drifting and the skillful restoration of conditions before that drift becomes damage.

Chronic illness rarely appears overnight. It arrives after a long conversation between the body and its circumstances, one that was legible long before the diagnosis was made. The patient who says "it came out of nowhere" almost always, on careful questioning, has a year or more of early signals behind the acute event. Lighter sleep. Less tolerant digestion. Slower recovery. More reactive moods. A body quietly narrowing.

We've seen this so often that it has become one of the first things we listen for in an intake: not just "when did this start?" but "when did you first notice something was different?" The answer is almost always earlier than the patient expects, and that earlier window is often where the real story lives.

To read those signals and act on them is not to over-medicalize ordinary life. It is to respect the timeline that chronic illness actually follows, and to intervene when doing so still makes sense.

THE TRIGGER IS NOT THE WHOLE STORY

The fourth argument is one that chronic illness makes unavoidable, even when acute medicine finds it difficult to accommodate.

Two people are exposed to the same virus. One recovers in a week. The other does not recover for months: lingering fatigue, dysregulation, a body that seems unable to complete the arc of illness and return to baseline. Two people experience the same loss. One metabolizes grief over time and emerges changed but functional. The other enters a years-long spiral of sleep disruption, inflammatory flares, and hormonal instability.

The external trigger is identical. The outcome diverges completely. And that divergence, the difference in terrain, in reserve, in regulatory capacity, in the body's ability to mount a response and then resolve it, is where most of chronic illness actually lives.

We explored this in the chapters on constitution and temporality. Modern medicine is extraordinarily good at identifying and eliminating external threats: pathogens, tumors, allergens, toxins. Chinese medicine is particularly oriented toward the internal terrain. Not because external threats don't matter, but because the terrain determines how the body responds to them. A well-resourced, well-regulated system can tolerate the same insults that collapse a depleted one, and the difference between those two outcomes is not moral. It's physiological.

This changes what we treat. Identifying the trigger, though important, is rarely sufficient. The body may have long since stopped responding to the original trigger and begun responding to the pattern it adopted in trying to survive it. Remember the microphone feedback loop from Chapter 1: the screech sustains itself long after the original sound has disappeared.

What the body is doing now, in response to a pattern it learned then, is the clinical material. Not the original insult, which may be irretrievable or irrelevant, but the current organization of compensation and exhaustion and misplaced vigilance that has become the person's baseline.

And that baseline can change. Not always completely, not always quickly, but the internal terrain is more responsive to skilled intervention than it appears from the outside, especially when the intervention is matched to the actual pattern rather than to the original cause.

HEALTH IS A RANGE, NOT A STATE

The fifth argument is perhaps the most quietly radical, because it proposes a different definition of what we are trying to achieve.

If health is the absence of symptoms, then treatment ends when the symptoms disappear. Success is silence. The body returns to neutral, and medicine steps back.

But you know from your own life, or from the clinic, that symptoms can be absent while everything essential is brittle. A person can be technically "fine" (normal labs, no active diagnosis, nothing diagnosable) and still be a single bad night of sleep away from a collapse. Still unable to travel without digestive disruption. Still requiring pharmaceutical assistance to fall asleep and still flaring with any deviation from a very narrow dietary range. Still held together by compensations that are working, but one major stressor away from failing.

That kind of stability isn't health in any meaningful sense. It's a system maintaining appearances while the margin keeps shrinking. And if our definition of health doesn't account for that distinction, we end up discharging people into a state of fragility and calling it success.

Health, as this medicine understands it, is closer to adaptability than to silence. It is the body's capacity to handle variation (dietary, climatic, emotional, physical) and return to equilibrium without catastrophe. The ability to exert and recover. To feel and settle. To get sick and get well. To absorb disruption without reorganizing your entire life around it.

When you hold that definition, it becomes what treatment is actually for. Not the eradication of every symptom, which is often impossible and sometimes inadvisable, but the recovery of enough flexibility that the body can meet ordinary life without crisis. It's what allows someone to live a full life rather than a managed one. To go to the dinner party without anxiety about the menu. To handle the difficult conversation without being derailed for three days. To catch a cold and recover rather than falling into a two-week spiral.

This is also, honestly, a more achievable goal than perfect health as usually imagined. The question shifts from "are you cured?" to "are you more capable than you were?" And that shift creates a different relationship to the slow, nonlinear nature of chronic healing, where progress sometimes looks like better recovery from a flare, not the elimination of flares altogether. Where success sometimes looks like digestion that handles stress with mild protest instead of a three-day collapse. Where improvement sometimes looks like sleeping through the night on most nights, not every night.

These aren't consolation prizes. They're real changes in a real system, accumulated over real time, and they compound. A body that is slightly more adaptive this month becomes more adaptive next month. The range expands. Options return. And at some point, the person stops thinking of themselves as fragile, which changes everything about how they move through their life.

None of This Belongs to Chinese Medicine Alone

Systems biology is arriving at similar conclusions through its own methods, moving away from single causes and toward networks, away from suppressing dysfunction and toward understanding it, away from disease categories and toward individual terrain. The intellectual arc of modern biomedicine, at its most sophisticated, bends in exactly this direction.

What the classical tradition offers is not a competing ideology. It is a several-thousand-year head start, an accumulated record of what these principles look like when applied daily with actual people, in all their messiness, variation, and refusal to behave like textbook cases.

That record is imperfect. The tradition contains errors, outdated assumptions, and sometimes confident claims that don't survive scrutiny. A good practitioner knows this and updates accordingly. The tradition itself, at its best, always expected that.

But underneath the terminology, underneath the historical context, underneath everything that requires translation, there is something durable: a coherent way of being with complexity. A willingness to stay in the room with a case that doesn't resolve cleanly. A set of questions that remain useful even when the answers remain partial.

CONCLUSION

There is a phrase we've heard in various forms from different teachers: "Treat the person, not the disease."

It can sound like a slogan until you sit with what it demands.

To treat the person is to accept that no two bodies express imbalance in exactly the same way. That the patient's story matters, not as decoration, but as diagnostic material and a map of what matters to them. That you can't fully separate physiology from life. That medicine is practiced in time, with feedback, with adjustment, with humility.

Chinese medicine, at its best, is an art not because it rejects rigor, but because it requires a kind of rigor that can't be reduced to checklists. Disciplined attention. Pattern recognition without rigidity. The courage to act without pretending to know everything, and the willingness to learn from the body in front of you, especially when it surprises you.

For the practitioner, the path is long. You will be wrong sometimes. You will miss things. You will have brilliant moments that fail to generalize, and simple treatments that unexpectedly change everything. If you stay honest, the medicine will train you. It will make you more careful with your certainty and more precise with your questions.

For the patient, the invitation is also demanding, but in a different way. It asks you to participate. Not perfectly, not anxiously, but steadily. To notice what your body is doing. To allow that healing may be a process of regaining adaptability rather than achieving a fixed ideal.

Medicine, at its most honest, has never been about mastering the body. It has been about learning to read what the body is already doing, and having the skill and the restraint to work with that intelligence rather than against it.

When it works, it doesn't feel like magic. It feels like something older and more reliable: the system begins to make better decisions. The body becomes less trapped in its loops. The person regains options: sleep, appetite, calm, movement and resilience. Life becomes less negotiated around symptoms and more lived on its own terms.

The medicine was never the needles, the herbs, or the terminology. It was always the quality of attention brought to bear on a person who needed to be seen clearly and treated as though their body made sense.

www.ingramcontent.com/pod-product-compliance
Ingram Content Group UK Ltd.
Pitfield, Milton Keynes, MK11 3LW, UK
UKHW022026190726
13853UKWH00005B/2136

9 798991 911399